# CHI SELF-MASSAGE

## The Taoist Way of Rejuvenation

*I have come upon Master Chia's Taoist prac-
tice in my old age and find it the most satis-
fying and enriching practice of all those I
have encountered in a long life of seeking and
practicing.*

—Felix Morrow
Healing Tao Books

# CHI SELF-MASSAGE

## The Taoist Way of Rejuvenation

# MANTAK CHIA

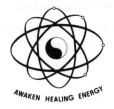

AWAKEN HEALING ENERGY

HEALING TAO BOOKS/HUNTINGTON, NEW YORK

First published in 1986 by
Healing Tao Books
P.O. Box 1194
Huntington, NY 11743

ISBN 0-935621-01-6
Library of Congress Card Number:
85-82051

Manufactured in the United States of America

03  04  05 / 15 14 13

# Contents

*Acknowledgments*     11

*A Word of Caution*     12

*About Master Mantak Chia*     13

*Author's Note*     17

**1. Benefits and Theory**     19

    I. Strong Senses Can Help Control Negative
       Emotions     20

    II. Healthy Organs Can Help to Change Emotional
       and Personal Characteristics     21

**2. The Anus Is Connected To Organ Energy**     23

    I. Perineum Power     24

    II. The Anus Region is Divided into Five Parts     25

    A. The middle part     26

    B. The front part     28

    C. The back part     29

    D. The left part     30

    E. The right part     32

**3. The Healing Hand**     35

    I. The Palms     36

    II. The Pericardium     36

    III. The Large Intestine     36

    IV. The Major Palm Lines     38

    V. The Fingers Have Corresponding Bodily Functions     38

   VI. Strengthen the Extremities      40

  VII. Massage the Hands to Increase the Flow of Chi   41

 VIII. Preparation

   IX. Practice   42

     A. Bring Chi energy to the hands   42

     B. Massage the hands   44

    X. The Fingers Correspond to Emotions, Elements   48
       and Organs

## 4. The Head Massage   51

    I. Head   53

     A. Crown point   53

     B. Bring Chi energy to the hands and face   54

     C. Knock the head   54

     D. Hold your breath to increase Chi flow   55

     E. Scalp   55

     F. Crest   56

   II. Face   56

     A. Natural beauty   56

     B. Bring Chi energy to the face   57

     C. Forehead   58

     D. Mid-face   60

     E. Lower face   60

     F. Whole face   60

     G. Mid-forehead   61

  III. Temples   62

  IV. Mouth   62

     A. Beautify the mouth massage   63

   V. Eyes   64

     A. Bring Chi energy to the hands and eyes   64

     B. For the eyeballs and surrounding area   66

     C. Pull up the eyelids   67

     D. For the eye sockets   67

    E.  For getting a tear out                              68

    F.  Pull in the eyeballs                                69

    G.  Learn to maintain eye contact                       72

  VI.  Nose                                                 72

    A.  Bring Chi energy to the hands                       73

    B.  Nostrils                                            73

    C.  Bridge                                              74

    D.  Mid-nose                                            75

    E.  Sides of the nose                                   75

    F.  Lower nose                                          76

 VII.  Ears                                                 76

    A.  Outer ear                                           77

    B.  Inner ear                                           79

VIII.  Gums, Tongue, Teeth                                  82

    A.  Bring Chi energy to the hands                       82

    B.  Gums                                                82

    C.  Gums and tongue                                     82

    D.  Tongue                                              84

    E.  Teeth clenching                                     85

    F.  Energy to teeth                                     86

  IX.  Neck                                                 87

    A.  Thyroid and parathyroid: the site of courage,
        the power of speech                                 87

    B.  Bring Chi energy to the hands                       89

    C.  Whole neck                                          89

    D.  Middle neck                                         89

    E.  Turtle neck                                         90

    F.  Crane neck                                          90

    G.  Massage the neck                                    91

   X.  Shoulders                                            92


**5.  Detoxifying Organs and Glands**                       95

    I.  Thymus Gland                                        96

|  |  |
|---|---|
| II. Heart | 97 |
| III. Lungs | 98 |
| IV. Liver | 98 |
| V. Stomach, Spleen, Pancreas | 98 |
| VI. Large and Small Intestines | 100 |
| VII. Kidneys | 102 |
| VIII. Sacrum | 103 |

## 6. Knees and Feet

105

| I. Knees Are Toxin Collectors, Too | 106 |
|---|---|
| A. Bring Chi energy to the hands | 106 |
| B. Behind the knees | 106 |
| C. Knee cap massage | 107 |
| D. Move the knee cap | 107 |
| E. Massage the knees | 107 |
| II. Feet, the Roots of the Body | 108 |
| A. Bring Chi energy to the hands | 108 |
| B. Massage the feet | 109 |
| C. Spread out the toes | 110 |
| D. Big and second toes | 110 |
| E. Rub feet together | 110 |

## 7. Constipation

111

| I. A Major Cause of Stress | 112 |
|---|---|
| II. Constipation Causes Holding Back and Lack of Openness | 112 |
| III. Constipation Makes You Age Faster | 113 |
| IV. Abdominal Massage—the Wonder of Healing | 113 |
| A. Sleep face up | 114 |
| B. Rub your hands until warm | 114 |
| C. Massage the small intestine | 114 |
| V. Massage During Bowel Movements | 116 |

## 8. Daily Practice 119

    I. Warm Up in the Morning 120

    II. Check Your Energy Level Each Day 122

    III. Start With the Inner Smile 122

    IV. Clean Out the Blocked Energy Every Day 124

    V. Clean Out Yesterday's Toxins 124

    VI. Increase Lower Limb Circulation 127

    VII. Activate Vein Circulation 128

    VIII. Stretch the Tendons 129

    IX. Stretch the Neck and Spine Tendons 132

    X. Clean the Nine Openings 132

      A. The front door—the sexual opening 132

      B. The back door—the nutrients opening 134

      C. The seven windows 134

      D. Routine large intestine cleaning 134

    XI. Clean Out the Parts of the Face 135

      A. Eyes 135

      B. Nose 135

      C. Teeth 137

      D. Ears 137

      E. Neck 137

      F. Massage the head and comb the hair 137

    XII. Massage the Feet 137

    XIII. Look at Yourself in the Mirror 138

    XIV. Clean Water As a Cleanser 139

    XV. Utilize Your Time 140

      A. Find time to practice 140

      B. Sleepiness while driving 140

      C. Computer operators and desk workers 140

      D. Watching television 141

      E. Boots 141

      F. Evening practice 141

XVI.  Commuting Exercises                               141

XVII.  Sleep Position                                   143

XVII.  "Oh, No! Not Another Obligation!"                144

## The International Healing Tao System  . . . . . . .  Catalog 1-30

The Goal of the Taoist Practice
International Healing Tao Course Offerings
Outline of the Complete System of the Healing Tao
Course Descriptions:
    Introductory Level I: Awaken Healing Light
    Introductory Level II: Development of Internal Power
    Introductory Level III: The Way of Radiant Health
    Intermediate Level: Foundations of Spiritual Practice
    Advance Level: The Realm of Soul and Spirit

# ACKNOWLEDGMENTS

I thank foremost those Taoist Masters who were kind enough to share their knowledge with me, never imagining it would eventually be taught to Westerners. I acknowledge special thanks to Dena Saxer for seeing the need for this book to be published and for her encouragement and hard work on the initial manuscript.

I thank the many contributors essential to the book's final form: Dena Saxer, for writing a portion of this book, especially the basic step-by-step instructions, and for choosing the title; the artist, Juan Li, for spending many hours drawing and making illustrations of the body's internal functions and for his cover illustration; Gunther Weil, Rylin Malone, and many of my students for their feedback; Jo Ann Cutreria, our secretary, for making so many contacts and working endlessly; Daniel Bobek for long hours at the computer; John-Robert Zielinski for helping with the new computer system and for rearranging the files and programs to speed up the new process; Adam Sacks, our computer consultant, who assisted in solving computer problems as they arose during the final stages of production; Helen Stites for entering the text on the computer and for editing and proofreading; Valerie Meszaros for editing and for organizing the text into book form on the computer, proofreading and typesetting specification; and Cathy Umphress for design and paste ups. Special thanks are extended to Michael Winn for general editing; David Miller for design and overseeing production; and Felix Morrow for his valuable advice and help in producing the book. Felix Morrow has agreed to be the Publisher of Healing Tao Books.

Without my wife, Maneewan, and my son, Max, the book would have been academic—for their gifts, my gratitude and love.

## A Word Of Caution

The book does not give any diagnoses or suggestions for medication. It does provide a means to increase your strength and good health in order to overcome imbalances in your system. If there is illness, a medical doctor should be consulted.

# About
# Master Mantak Chia

Master Mantak Chia is the creator of the system known as The Healing Tao and is the Founder and Director of The Healing Tao Center in New York. Since childhood he has been studying the Tao way of life as well as other disciplines. The result of Master Chia's thorough knowledge of Taoism, enhanced by his knowledge of various other systems, is his development of The Healing Tao System, which is now being taught in many cities in the United States, Canada and Europe.

Master Chia was born in Thailand in 1944, and when he was six years old he learned to "sit and still the mind" (i.e., meditation) from Buddhist monks. While he was a grammar school student, he first learned traditional Thai boxing and then was taught Tai Chi Chuan by Master Lu, who soon introduced him to Aikido, Yoga and more Tai Chi.

Later, when he was a student in Hong Kong, excelling in track and field events, a senior classmate, Cheng Sue-Sue, presented him to his first esoteric teacher, Master Yi Eng, and he began his studies of the Taoist way of life. He learned how to pass life-force power from his hands, how to circulate energy through the Microcosmic Orbit, how to open the Six Special Channels, Fusion of the Five Elements, Enlightenment of the Kan and Li, Sealing of the Five Sense Organs,

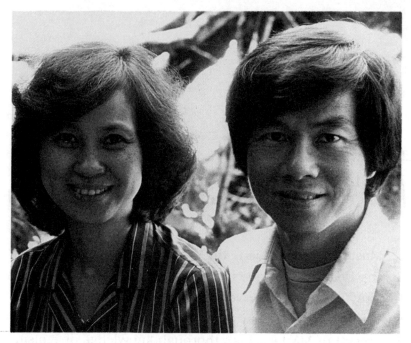

Mantak and Maneewan Chia

Congress of Heaven and Earth, and Reunion of Man and Heaven.

In his early twenties Mantak Chia studied with Master Meugi in Singapore, who taught him Kundalini Yoga and the Buddhist Palm, and he was soon able to eliminate blockages to the flow of life-force energy in his own body as well as in the patients of his Master.

In his later twenties he studied with Master Pan Yu, whose system combined Taoist, Buddhist and Zen teachings, and with Master Cheng Yao-Lun, whose system combined Thai boxing and Kung Fu. From Master Pan Yu he learned about the exchange of the Yin and Yang power between men and women and also the "steel body", a technique that keeps the body from decaying. Master Cheng Yao-Lun taught him the secret Shao-Lin Method of Internal

Power and the even more secret Iron Shirt method called Cleansing the Marrow and Renewal of the Tendons.

Then, to better understand the mechanisms behind the healing energy, Master Chia studied Western medical science and anatomy for two years. While pursuing his studies, he managed the Gestetner Company, a manufacturer of office equipment, and became well acquainted with the technology of offset printing and copying machines.

Using his knowledge of the complete system of Taoism as the foundation, and building onto that with what he learned from his other studies, he developed The Healing Tao System and began teaching it to others. He then trained teachers to assist him, and established The Natural Healing Center in Thailand. Five years later he decided to move to New York to introduce his system to the West, and in 1979 he opened The Healing Tao Center here. Since then, centers have been established in many other cities, including Boston, Philadelphia, Denver, Seattle, San Francisco, Los Angeles, San Diego, Tucson, Toronto, London and Bonn, among others.

Master Chia leads a peaceful life with his wife Maneewan, who teaches Taoist Five Element Nutrition at the New York Center, and their young son. He is a warm, friendly, and helpful man, who views himself primarily as a teacher. He uses a word processor when writing his books and is equally at ease with the latest computer technology as he is with esoteric philosophies.

He currently has written and published three Healing Tao Books: in 1983, *Awaken Healing Energy Through The Tao;* in 1984, *Taoist Secrets Of Love: Cultivating Male Sexual Energy;* and in 1985, *Taoist Ways to Transform Stress Into Vitality.* This book is his fourth volume.

## AUTHOR'S NOTE

In the last pages of this book, the reader will find descriptions of the courses and workshops offered by our Healing Tao Centers. This material is also in effect a comprehensive description of the whole Taoist system. All of my books together will be a composite of this Taoist world-view. Each of my books is thus an exposition of one important part of this system. Each sets forth a method of healing and life-enrichment which can be studied and practiced by itself, if the reader so chooses. Certainly, each is comprehensible by itself, but in the Taoist System, each of these methods implies the others and is best practiced in combination with the others. Thus, the foundation of all of them, the practice of the meditation of the Microcosmic Orbit, which is the way to circulate the Chi energy throughout our body, is involved in all the other practices. My book that is basically concerned with the Microcosmic Orbit is *Awaken Healing Energy.*

Two practices that follow are the meditation of the Inner Smile and the Six Healing Sounds. These, too, are also constantly emphasized. They are set forth in my book, *Taoist Ways to Transform Stress into Vitality.* The present book follows from all that has gone before it, but you can begin with this book and learn from it the full range of Chi self-massage. I do believe that once you begin to practice this network of Taoist Rejuvenation, it will create in you the desire to master the others that I have named. You will then be in a position to benefit fully from my book, *Taoist Secrets of Love: Cultivating Male Sexual Energy.* That is as far as my books have come. Concerning the others that will follow, I refer you again to the description of our courses and workshops.

*Mantak Chia*

# 1
# Benefits
# and
# Theory

From ancient times to the present, Taoist Masters have been remarkably youthful, appearing and functioning at least twenty years younger than their actual ages. One source of their vitality has been the practice of Taoist Self-Massage Rejuvenation: using one's internal energy, or Chi, to strengthen and rejuvenate the sense organs (eyes, ears, nose, tongue, teeth, skin) and the inner organs. These techniques are about five thousand years old and until now were closely guarded secrets passed on from one Master to a small group of students. Even so, each Master often knew only part of the method. Based on my studies with a number of different Taoist Masters, I have pieced together the entire method and organized the material into a logical routine. By practicing this routine five to ten minutes daily, you can improve many things, including your complexion, vision, hearing, sinuses, gums, teeth, tongue, and general stamina.

## I. Strong Senses Can Help Control Negative Emotions.

Self-Massage Rejuvenation works by clearing blockages from the meridians, or energy channels, of the various senses and vital organs. This is done by the unique Taoist practice of bringing energy, or Chi, up from the sexual organs and anus to the face, hands and senses, and then directing it to specific areas. The senses are connected with the organs, and the organs are believed to store and generate positive and negative emotions. By strengthening the senses, we help to control negative emotions. Senses are the first to receive the influences of the outside world, such as tension, anger and fear; and, in turn, these outside negative influences affect the organs and the nervous system. Strong senses will help to prevent an overload of outside influences that can negatively affect us.

## *II. Healthy Organs Can Help to Change Emotional and Personal Characteristics.*

In my ten years of teaching this simple self-massage, I have seen people use it to improve their emotional, personal and social lives. One of my students had strong fears which easily brought on anger. This resulted in moodiness, irritability and pain in his stomach. Feeling this way, a person is unlikely to be sociable, friendly or easy to communicate with. After a few weeks of practicing the Inner Smile, Liver Sound, and massaging the liver and stomach, this person's disposition improved, the moodiness decreased and he became friendlier. He says that since he began studying with me, the greatest benefit has been in his family life, especially his relationship with his children. Now he no longer needs to use the alcohol he relied upon to cover up his pain and forget the stress which previously affected him. His employer and co-workers also notice the change, and he has sent other workers to study the system.

I have a secretary who once paid for one of her co-workers to study with us, wanting her co-worker to find a way to better cope with stress on the job. This woman told me that it was the best investment she had ever made, because she no longer had to be victimized by her co-worker's emotional swings when they worked together.

# 2
# The Anus
# Is Connected To
# Organ Energy

In Tao Rejuvenation the Chi flow is very important. Without bringing Chi circulation to the part that you massage, it is just a simple, normal touch or massage. The Inner Smile and Microcosmic Orbit Meditation are very important also. They are the best ways to increase the life-force in the senses and organs.

## I. Perineum Power

The perineum (Hin-yin) region includes the anus and sexual organs. The anus region is divided into various sections which are closely linked to the Chi of corresponding organs. The Chinese term Hin-yin (perineum) means the collection point of all the Yin energy, or the lowest abdominal energy collection point. It is also known as the gate of death and life. This point lies between the two main gates. One we call the front gate (the sexual organ) which is the big life-force opening. Here the life-force energy can easily leak out and deplete the organ's function. The second gate, or back gate, is the anus. This gate can also easily lose life-force when not sealed or closed tight. In the Tao practices, especially in the Tao Secrets of Love, Healing Love and Iron Shirt, the perineum's power to tighten, close and draw the life-force back up the spine is an important practice. Otherwise, our life-force and sexual energy can become a "river of no return"; they will flow out and will not recycle back.

## II. The Anus Region is Divided into Five Parts.

The anus is divided into five regions: (A) middle, (B) front, (C) back, (D) left, and (E) right. (Figure 2–1)

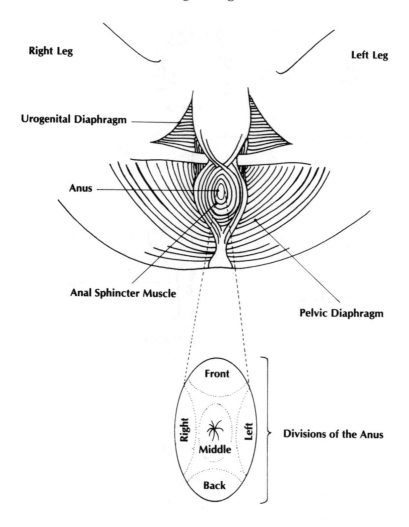

**Figure 2–1**

The anus is divided into five regions.

## A. The middle part

The middle of the anus Chi is connected with the organs as follows: the vagina-uterus, the aorta and vena cava, stomach, heart, thyroid and parathyroid glands, pituitary gland, pineal gland and the top of the head. (Figures 2–2 and 2–3)

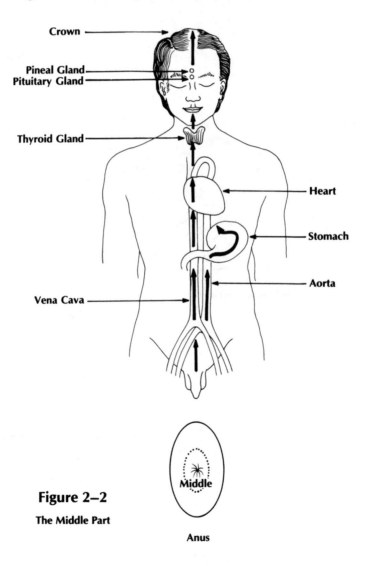

Crown

Pineal Gland
Pituitary Gland

Thyroid Gland

Heart

Stomach

Aorta

Vena Cava

Middle

Anus

**Figure 2–2**

**The Middle Part**

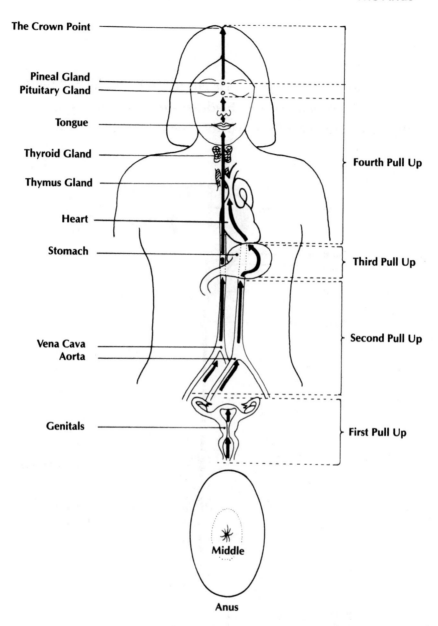

The Crown Point

Pineal Gland
Pituitary Gland

Tongue

Thyroid Gland

Thymus Gland

Heart

Stomach

Vena Cava
Aorta

Genitals

Fourth Pull Up

Third Pull Up

Second Pull Up

First Pull Up

Middle

Anus

**Figure 2–3**

## B. The front part

The front of the anus Chi is connected with the following organs: the prostate gland, bladder, small intestine, stomach, thymus gland, and front part of the brain. (Figure 2–4)

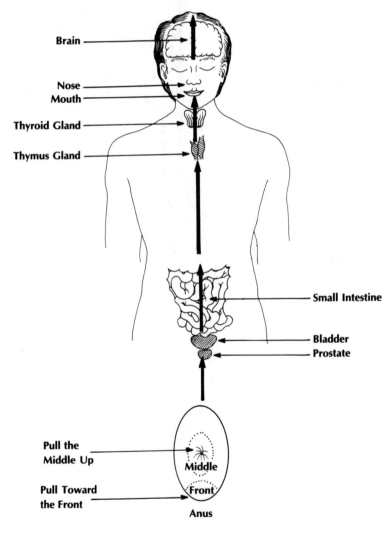

**Figure 2–4**

**The Front Part**

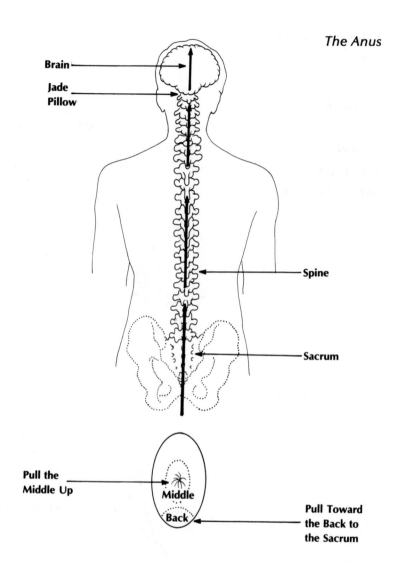

**Figure 2–5**

The Back Part

## C. The back part

The back part of the anus Chi is connected with the organ energies of: the sacrum, lower lumbars, the twelve thoracic vertebrae, the seven cervical vertebrae, and the small brain (cerebellum). (Figure 2–5)

## D. The left part

The left part of the anus Chi is connected with the organ energies of: the left ovary, the large intestine, left kidney, adrenal gland, spleen, left lung and left hemisphere of the brain. (Figures 2–6 and 2–7)

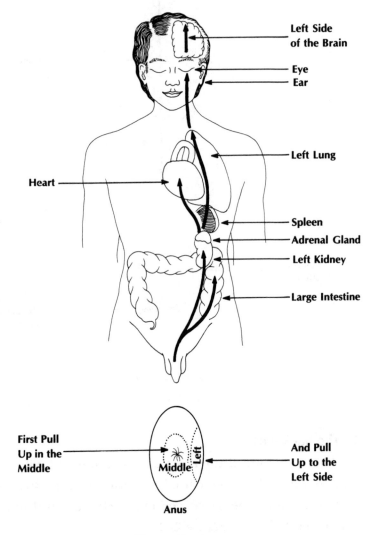

**Figure 2–6**

**The Left Part In the Male**

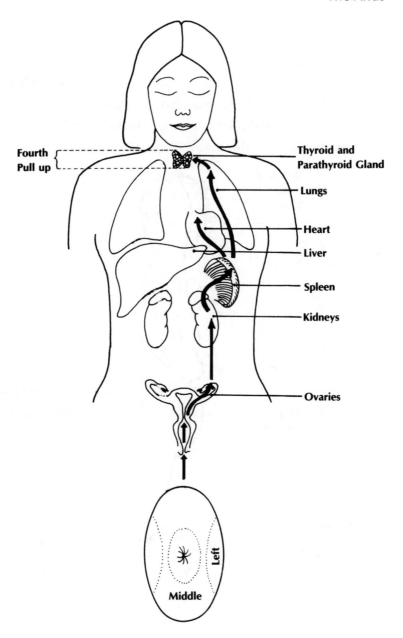

**Figure 2–7**

**The Left Part In the Female**

### E. The right part

The right part of the anus Chi is connected with the organ energies as follows: the right ovary, the large intestine, right kidney, adrenal gland, liver, gall bladder, right lung and right hemisphere of the brain. (Figure 2-8)

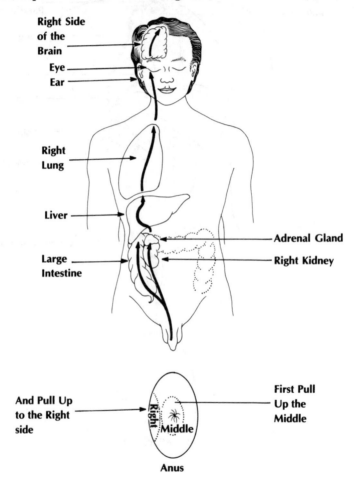

**Figure 2–8**

**The Right Part in the Male**

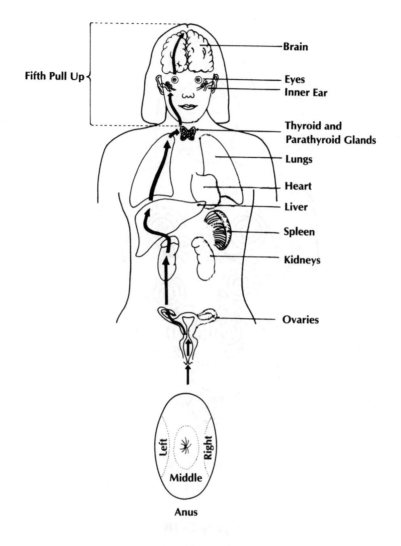

**Figure 2–9**

The Right Part in the Female

By contracting the different parts of the anus, you can bring more Chi to the organs and glands, and the effects of the massage will increase. (Figures 2–9 and 2–10)

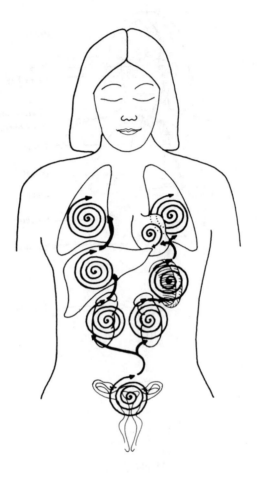

**Figure 2–10**

Drop and circle the energy around the organs.

# 3
# The
# Healing
# Hand

Humans can build all kinds of sophisticated instruments because of the magnificence of the hands and the fingers. Another higher function of the hands is the power of healing. Knowing the major points of the hands and fingers will enable you to stimulate and maintain the organs in good function.

## I. The Palms

The palms are where all major energies of Chi join. The palm can be the place from which the life-force is sent out to heal others or yourself. The palm also is the place where energy can be received and enter into the bone structure and into the major organs.

## II. The Pericardium

The pericardium (P–8) is the main place of energy concentration. You can collect the energy in this point and transmit stronger energy from this point. (Figure 3–1)

## III. The Large Intestine

The large intestine (LI–4) is the major point which controls all the pain in the body, especially in the sense organs (eyes, ears, nose) and headaches. (Figure 3-2)

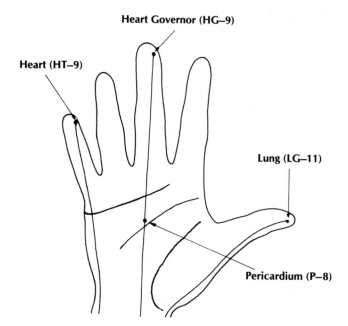

**Figure 3–1**

The Pericardium

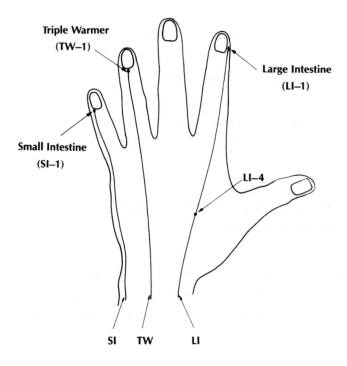

**Figure 3–2**

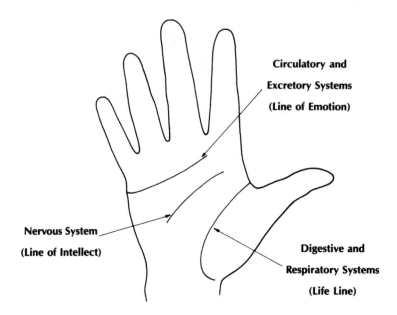

Circulatory and
Excretory Systems
(Line of Emotion)

Nervous System
(Line of Intellect)

Digestive and
Respiratory Systems
(Life Line)

**Figure 3–3**

The Three Major Palm Lines

## IV. The Major Palm Lines

The three major palm lines are the Life Line, the Line of Intellect and the Line of Emotion. (Figure 3–3)

## V. The Fingers Have Corresponding Bodily Functions.

The fingers are connected to the organs' meridians. (Figure 3–4) The joints of the finger bones are also related to parts of the organs and their corresponding senses and emotions.

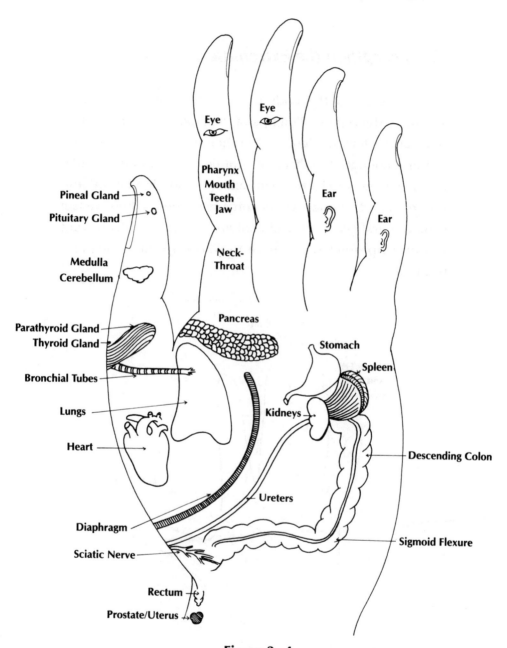

## Figure 3–4

**The Fingers and Their Corresponding Bodily Functions
Through the Organs' Meridians**

## VI. Strengthen the Extremities.

Strengthening the ends of the extremities will help to stimulate the organs. The tips of the fingers have many tiny veins and arteries. (Figure 3–5) When we get old and do not exercise enough, the Chi does not flow well and its circulation becomes stuck. This can affect blood circulation, and the veins and arteries will become hardened. When we feel cool, the first places to feel cool are the hands. If you want to warm up quickly, you have to warm up the hands and feet first.

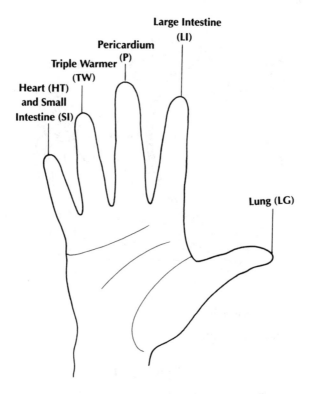

**Figure 3–5**

**Strengthening the ends of the extremities will help to stimulate the organs.**

## VII.  Massage the Hands to Increase the Flow of Chi.

Massaging the hands and palms will help to increase the flow of Chi along the related meridians and will result in a harmonious increase of the functions of respiration, circulation and digestion.

## VIII.  Preparation

A. Wait at least an hour after eating.

B. Try this practice immediately after doing the Inner Smile or Six Healing Sounds.* For the best results, if you have already learned the Microcosmic Orbit or Fusion Meditations, try this technique after practicing these as well.

C. Sit comfortably on your sitting bones at the edge of a chair. Make sure that your legs are grounded. Loosen your belt. Remove your glasses, watch and shoes.

D. In general, massage each area six to nine times. Massage problem areas more.

E. Those people who cannot get out of bed can practice the routine there.

* For a complete exposition of the Inner Smile and the Six Healing Sounds, see the author's preceding book, *Taoist Ways to Transform Stress Into Vitality.*

## IX. Practice

### A. Bring Chi energy to the hands. (Figure 3-6)

1. Inhale, contract your vagina or testicles, your buttocks, and also the part of the anus which is named—that is, the front, back, right, left, middle, or entire anus. At first you may not be sensitive to these distinctions, but eventually you will be. In general, the part of the anus which is contracted corresponds to the location of the area to be massaged. For example, you contract the left side of the anus when massaging the left lung.

2. Hold your breath and hold the contractions, clench your teeth together, and press your tongue to the roof of your mouth, as you rub your hands together vigorously. This stimulates the twelve meridians in the hands.

3. Continue to rub your hands while holding your breath and contracting your anus. Feel your face getting hot. Then, mentally picture energy flowing to your hands.

4. When your face and hands are hot, direct your attention to the appropriate area and massage that part until you are out of breath. Exhale and breathe normally. Smile and become aware of the part that is being massaged. Feel that the area is exceptionally warm and that energies are flowing.

5. Repeat this entire procedure for each area to be massaged or whenever your hands become cool. Your hands must always be very warm for self-massage. Cold hands will have very little effect on the massage.

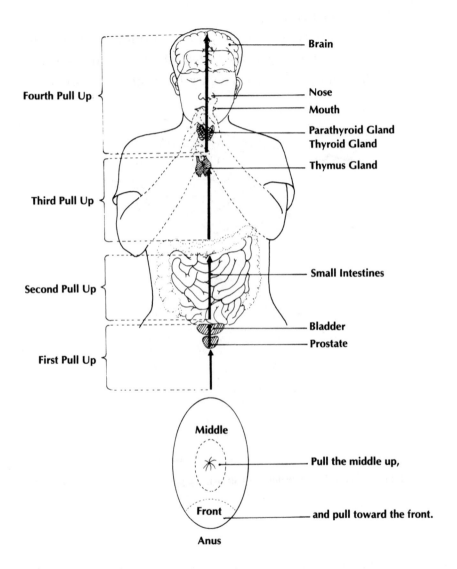

Fourth Pull Up

Third Pull Up

Second Pull Up

First Pull Up

Brain

Nose

Mouth

Parathyroid Gland
Thyroid Gland

Thymus Gland

Small Intestines

Bladder

Prostate

Middle

Front

Anus

Pull the middle up,

and pull toward the front.

## Figure 3–6

**Bringing Chi Energy to the Hands**

## B. Massage the hands.

Always start by rubbing your hands until they are warm.

1. Massage the pericardium (P–8). Use the thumb to press the middle of the palm with a circular motion. (Figure 3–7)

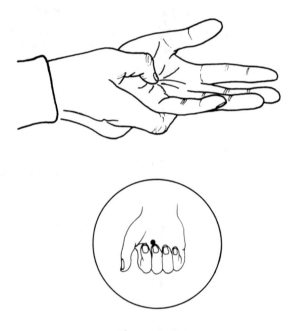

**Figure 3–7**

**Massaging the Pericardium**

**With fingers cupped in the palm in a half-fist, the pericardium is the point at the tip of the middle finger.**

2. Massage the hegu (LI-l4). Press the thumb around the point in a circular motion, and press more at the index finger bone. Find the pain point and massage it away. (Figure 3-8)

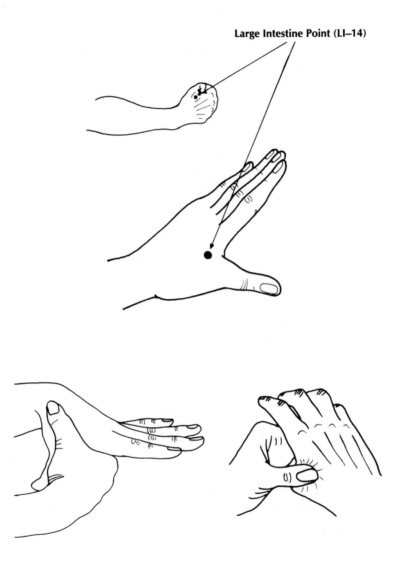

**Large Intestine Point (LI–14)**

**Figure 3–8**

Massaging LI–14

3. Massage the major palm lines. Use the thumb to massage along the palm lines. Massage more towards the thumb bone and along that bone. When a lot of emotion is held inside, find the sore point and massage it. (Figure 3–9)

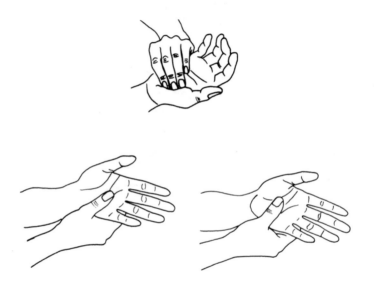

**Figure 3–9**

**Massaging the Palm Lines**

4. Massage the back of the hand. Use the thumb to press along the bones on the back of the hand. When you find a tender spot, take more time to work on it. (Figure 3–10)

5. Massage the fingers. Always rub your hands until warm. Use the right hand's fingers to wrap around the left thumb, and then, one by one, squeeze, hold and release each

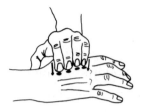

**Figure 3–10**

Massage the back of the hand

finger on the left hand three to six times. Start with the left hand and continue to the right hand's fingers, according to the elements of the finger. This will greatly help to control emotions. (Figure 3–11)

For example, if at any time you are frightened or fearful, you can wrap your fingers around the little finger, starting with the left side and moving to the right side. This can be a great help when you are in a difficult situation, such as talk-

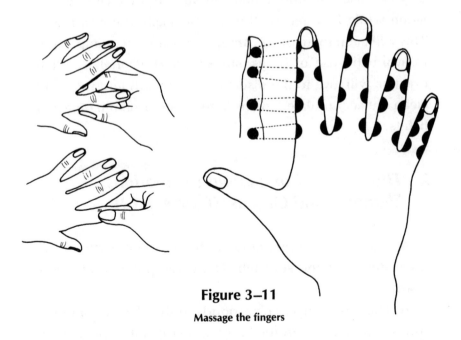

**Figure 3–11**

Massage the fingers

ing before a group of people, going on an interview, or meeting important people. Practicing the Heart and Kidney Sounds in conjunction with the finger wrapping may also help. The ring finger controls anger; when you are going to get angry, try to wrap it a few times to see if you still get angry.

Daily practice of the Inner Smile and the Six Healing Sounds is the best way to gain control of negative emotions. Many students are addicted to smoking, drugs or alcohol. The toxic elements found in these substances settle in the organs and nervous system, stimulating them into overactivity, and in a short period of time make people high. When the effect is over, the users will start to feel low key energy, becoming emotional and nervous. In this situation, they can use the Inner Smile and Microcosmic Orbit circulation while holding the fingers, especially the ring finger. This will calm them down. Many people use this simple way to avoid the use of drugs, smoking and alcohol. The Tao practice will give to the disciple the strength and power to clean out accumulated toxins in the system, eliminating bad habits.

## X. The Fingers Correspond to Emotions, Elements and Organs. (Figure 3-12)

A. The thumb corresponds to the element earth and is associated with the stomach. The corresponding emotion is worry.

B. The index finger corresponds to the element of metal and is associated with the lungs and large intestine. It links with the emotions of sadness, grief and depression.

C. The middle finger corresponds with the element of fire and is associated with the heart, small intestine, circulatory system and the respiratory system. It links with the emotions of impatience and hastiness.

D. The ring finger corresponds to the wood element and is associated with the liver, gall bladder and the nervous system; it corresponds to the anger emotion.

E. The little finger corresponds to the water element; it is associated with the kidneys, and corresponds with the emotion of fear.

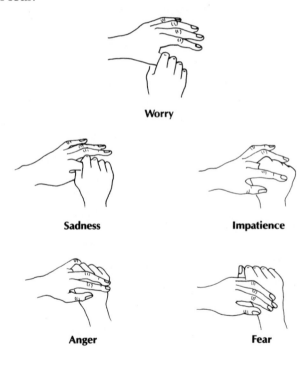

**Figure 3–12**

**The fingers' corresponding emotions, elements and organs.**

# 4
# The
# Head
# Massage

The head massage is for headaches, nervousness, and an imbalance of Chi energy in the brain.

The causes of headaches and nervousness are very complex. The head is the place in which all the nerves are seated and is the central control of the whole system. Nowadays you see a lot of young people who are very nervous. This nervousness causes insomnia, loss of appetite, faster heart beat, difficulty in breathing, tiredness, laziness, etc. It seems that all of this is not symptomatic, but it greatly affects the efficiency of work and gradually is considered mental disease.

The skull massage will strengthen the nervous system. With the tongue touching the roof of the mouth as it is during the massage, and the eyes moving up to the left and then across to the right, you can feel the stimulation of the Chi energy from left to right. This balances the left and right hemispheres of the brain and will result in strengthening the glands, senses and organs.

The head and skull massage will increase the blood circulation and will increase the nutrition of the skull and hair. We have students whose white hair grew black and students whose falling hair became denser as more hair grew back. The hair also grows softer. In the morning and at night before sleeping, you should brush your hair at least 25–50 times. Find a good brush, and be careful of the scalp. Do not scratch the skull, which might result in a headache or sense of pain.

## I. Head

### A. Crown point (Figure 4–1)

This is located in the center of the crown; in the fontanelle area of an infant's skull there may still be a slight depression. The crown point is the junction of one hundred channels through which the energy of the body passes. Massage this area with both your middle fingers. This will relieve dizziness and headaches, which result from too much energy in the head. It also relieves high blood pressure and stimulates the nervous system.

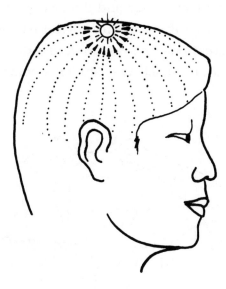

**Figure 4–1**

The Crown Point is the junction point of one hundred energy channels.

## B. Bring Chi energy to the hands and face.

Inhale, contract the sexual organ, buttocks, and middle of the anus. Rub the hands, clench the teeth, and put the tongue to the roof of the mouth. When the face, head, and hands are hot, breathe normally and begin to massage.

## C. Knock the head. (Figure 4-2)

Hit the head with the knuckles of the hand, knocking all around the head. Knocking the head lightly can help to clear your head, eliminate stubbornness and make your thinking sharper. Many of our students use this knocking of the head to release the pressures that they have from today's life of fast, advanced technology and the feeling of always having to keep up. This is especially true of those graduate students who feel a great deal of pressure and stress in keeping up with their studies. Each year students commit suicide be-

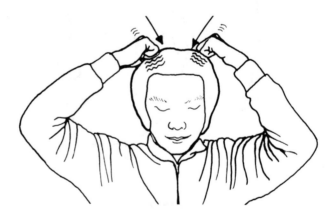

**Figure 4–2**

**Knocking the head**

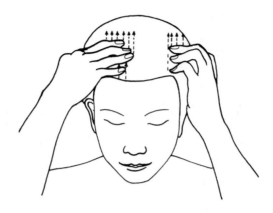

**Figure 4–3**

Massaging the scalp

cause the pressures and stress accumulate too much in their heads, making them unable to think clearly; they start to feel everything in their society as too much pressure, which leads to worry, fear, sadness, and many mixed emotions. The simple knocking of the head can release pressure and stress that accumulate there.

### D. Hold your breath to increase Chi flow.

Holding your breath will increase the Chi flow to the face. The head has many channels that join in the skull, especially in the crown point.

### E. Scalp (Figure 4-3)

Prepare your hands, head and scalp by warming up. Using both hands like a comb, press hard and move slowly, massage the scalp, going straight back from the hairline to the base of the skull. As you do this, mentally direct your energy from the back of the skull to your feet. Repeat 6–9 times. Massage more in any places in which you feel pain, until the pain goes away.

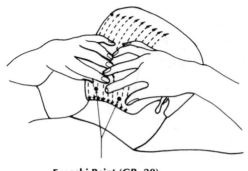

Fengchi Point (GB–20)

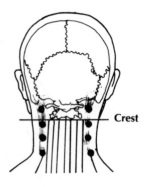

Crest

**Figure 4—4**

Crest, the edge of the skull

**Figure 4—5**

Go straight back from the
hairline to the base of the skull.

### F. Crest (Figure 4-4)

Using your thumbs, massage the crest (the edge) at the base of the skull until you feel no pain there. (Figure 4–5) This will help you reduce headaches and eye aches and will increase vision. This place in Tao tradition is called the Pool of Wind which tends to collect the "evil wind", the major cause of all the pain in the senses.

## II.  Face (Figures 4–6, 4–8 and 4–9)

### A. Natural Beauty

Massaging your face with Chi is a far more effective beauty treatment than the most expensive cream or cosmetic. (Figure 4–10) Your skin will glow brightly and eventually become less wrinkled. There are many meridians passing through or ending at the face. When blocked, they result in reduced flow of Chi energy and circulation. The face is the first impression imprinted in other people's minds. Chi circulation provides it with attractive personal energy.

## B. Bring Chi energy to the face.

Inhale, contract your sexual organ, buttocks, and middle and front of the anus. Hold your breath, rub your hands together, clench your teeth, and put your tongue to the roof of your mouth. When your face feels hot, picture energy flowing to your hands. When your hands are very warm, bring your attention to your face and hold your breath until your face gets hot.

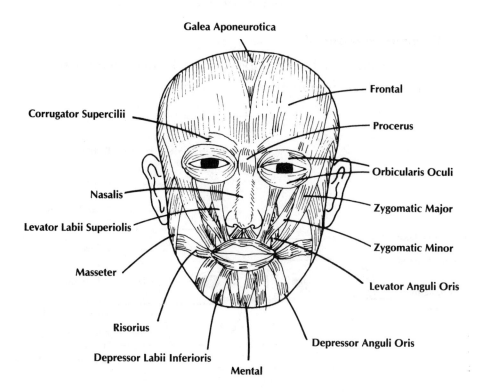

**Figure 4–6**

**The Facial Muscles**

57

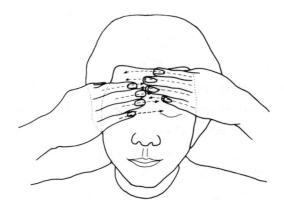

**Figure 4–7**

Wiping your forehead

## C. Forehead (Figure 4-7)

Using alternate hands, wipe your forehead from one side to the other six to nine times.

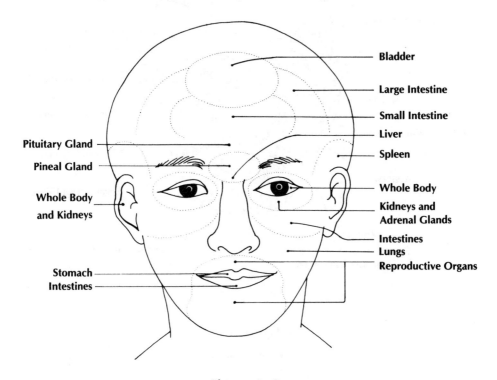

**Figure 4–8**

Diagrams of the Face Corresponding to the Organs

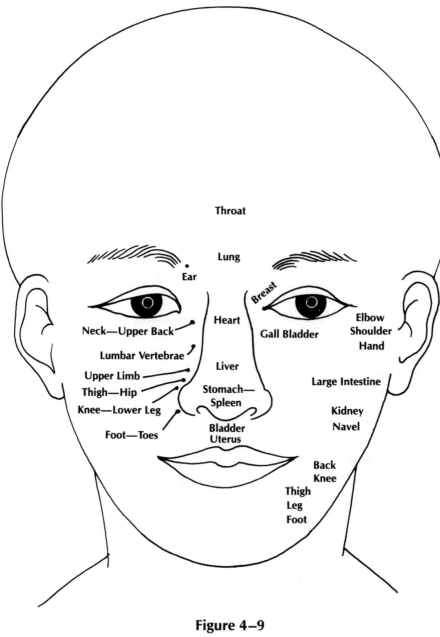

Figure 4–9

Head and Face

59

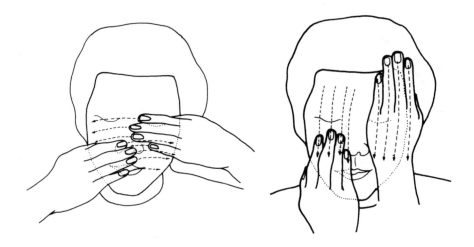

**Figure 4–10**

Your own Chi energy is the best cosmetic.

### D. Mid-face

Wipe the middle section of the face, from the eyebrows to the tip of your nose.

### E. Lower face

Repeat for the lower section of the face, below the nose to your chin.

### F. Whole face

Repeat the procedure for bringing energy to your hands. Inhale, cover your whole face with your palms and massage it. (Figure 4–11) Use an upward motion to reduce wrinkles. Exhale and relax your face. Rest and smile to your face until you can feel it tingle with warmth.

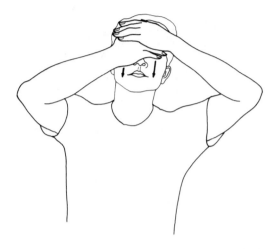

**Figure 4–11**

Massage the whole face.

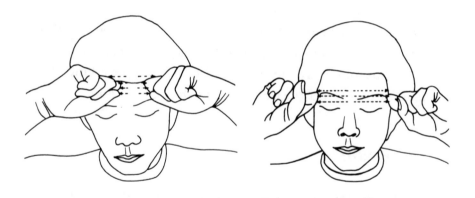

**Figure 4–12**

Massage the mid-forehead.

## G. Mid-forehead

Use the second joint of alternate index fingers to massage the middle of the forehead, from the center to the temple. (Figure 4–12)

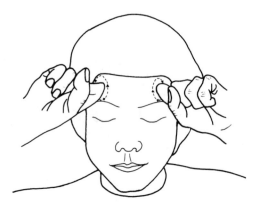

**Figure 4–13**

Massage the temples.

## III. Temples

Use your index fingers to massage the temples in a circular motion, first clockwise, then counterclockwise. Massage the forehead and the temples; use the knuckle rub from the middle of the forehead all the way to the temples ten to twenty times. (Figure 4–13) These exercises will reduce headaches in the front and in the temples. Find the painful point and massage it until the pain is gone.

## IV. Mouth

Depression makes the corners of the mouth drop. Looking cheerful, delightful, more attractive and happy are dependent so much on the eyes and the corners of the mouth. When the muscles of the mouth are loose because of stress, depression, or sadness, the corners of the mouth drop and the energy system is depressed and in low key. No one likes to look at a sad face or a depressed face; it makes other people feel sad and depressed, too.

The flow of energy in the body and the expression of the face are the main attractive powers of a person. Massaging the mouth muscles up will help to lift the corners of the mouth. The Inner Smile and lifting up the corners of the mouth are very important to building up attractive energy.

### A. Beautify the mouth massage

Using the thumb and the index finger of the right hand, touch both corners of the mouth and feel the Chi from the thumb and index finger pass to the corners of the mouth. Slowly press and push up about one inch, release and start again at the corners, pressing up ten to twenty times each day. (Figure 4–14)

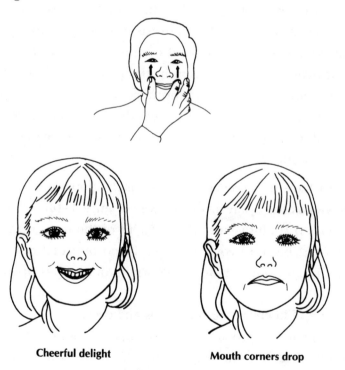

Cheerful delight          Mouth corners drop

**Figure 4–14**

Beautifying the mouth massage

## V. Eyes

The eyes are the windows of the spirit. (Figure 4–15) In Taoism we regard the eyes as Yang energy which will guide all Chi flow in the body. The eyes can greatly affect your personality. Some people are born with a lot of white in their eyes—three portions of white to one portion of iris—sometimes called "thief eyes" or "danger attack eyes." Such eyes can result in a suspicious look, portending unpleasant things. Through the exercises, you can gradually correct the white portion of the eyes.

Since the eyes are connected to the entire nervous system, they have a special importance. The eyes reveal the health of your entire body. Through the eyes we can tell which organs are weak and/or toxic. Massaging the eyes will remove stress from the vital organs. Nowadays people use their eyes much more than in the past to read, watch television, and work with computers, electronics and microscopes. This strains them a great deal and makes the openings of the organs loose, so that much of the organ energy is drained out.

In Taoism, we regard the eyes as the doorways to the soul as well as the opening of the liver. (Figure 4–16)

When rubbing near the corners of the eyes, do not rub too hard, because you can make the corners of the eyes drop down. Continue rubbing the corners of the eyes upward.

### A. Bring Chi energy to the hands and eyes.

Repeat the procedure for bringing energy to the hands by inhaling; holding the breath; and contracting the sexual organ, buttocks and middle of the anus and both the left and right sides of the anus. Direct the Chi to both eyes. Rub the hands, clench the teeth, place the tongue on the roof of your

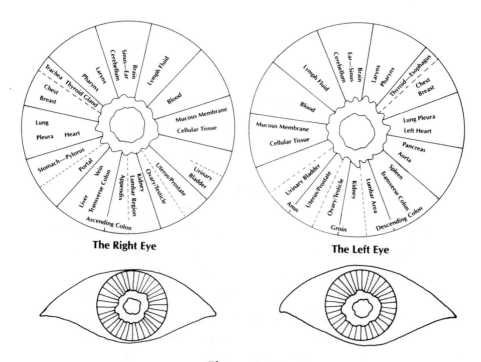

**The Right Eye**          **The Left Eye**

## Figure 4–15

The eyes are the windows of the spirit.

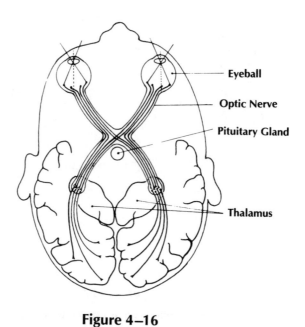

Eyeball

Optic Nerve

Pituitary Gland

Thalamus

## Figure 4–16

The eyes are the doorways to the soul.

65

mouth. Direct the energy to the face and then the hands. When your hands are hot, focus on your eyes until you feel them filled with energy.

### B. For the eyeballs and surrounding area

Close your eyes. Use your fingertips to gently massage your eyeballs through your closed eyelids, six to nine times clockwise, then six to nine times counterclockwise. Then gently massage the area around the lids the same number of times. (Figure 4–17) Be aware of painful spots and massage those places until the pain goes away. Pay special attention to the inner and outer corners of the eyes. These are points of the gall bladder meridian and will relieve eye ailments if massaged.

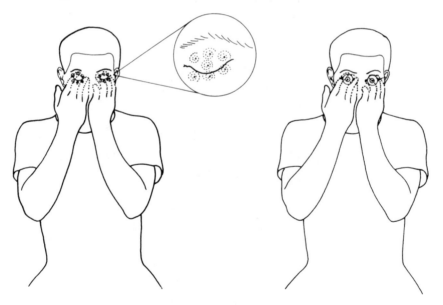

**Figure 4–17**

Use the fingertips to gently massage the eyeballs.

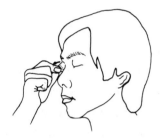

**Figure 4–18**

Pull up the eyelids.

## C. Pull up the eyelids.

Pulling up the eyelids will increase the fluid. Use the thumb and index finger to pinch, pull up and release the eyelids six to nine times. (Figure 4–18)

## D. For the eye sockets

Bend your index fingers and use the lower section (second phalanx) of each thumb to rub the upper and lower bones of the eye sockets six to nine times. (Figure 4–19)

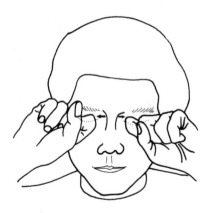

**Figure 4–19**

Massage the eye sockets.

### E. For getting a tear out

Hold an index finger up about eight inches from the eyes, or put a dot on the wall five or six feet away from you. Stare at it intently without blinking your eyes until you feel like a fire is burning in them. (Figure 4–20) The Taoists believe that the toxins will burn out of the body through the eyes. They will begin to tear. Do this to strengthen your eyes. Then, rub your hands until warm; close your eyes and cover your eye sockets with your palms. Feel the Chi from the hands absorbed into the eyes. (Figure 4–21) Rotate your eyes six to nine times, first in a clockwise direction, then counterclockwise.

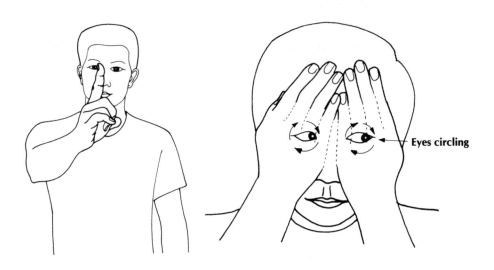

**Figure 4–20**

Getting a tear out

**Figure 4–21**

Absorbing the Chi into the eyes

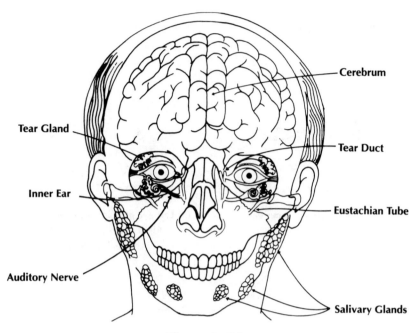

**Figure 4–22**

The parts of the eyes connect with the senses and brain.

## F. Pull in the eyeballs.

The eyes are divided into five parts. Each part is closely connected with the organs and nerves. (Figure 4–22) Become aware of the eyes. (Figure 4–23)

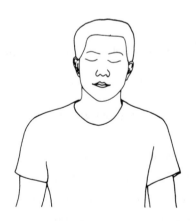

**Figure 4–23**

Awareness of the eyes

69

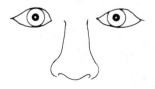

(1) Pressing into the inner ear

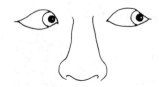

(2) Left eye pressing into the ear canal
Right eye pressing into the
eustachian tube

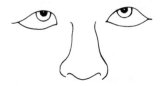

(3) Pressing into the pituitary gland

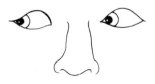

(4) Right eye pressing into the ear canal
Left eye pressing into the
eustachian tube

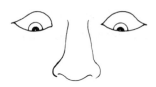

(5) Pressing into the eustachian tube

**Figure 4–24**

Pulling and pressing the eyeballs will exercise the organs, senses, glands and the brain. (Figures 4–24) This is also the best exercise for the eye muscles. The eyes have many muscles which we do not exercise very much and, thus, they become weak, contributing to poor eyesight.

1. With the eyes still closed and cupped by the palms, inhale, contract the anus and sexual organ, and pull the eyeballs back into the sockets.

2. Contract the middle of the anus and the middles of the eyeballs.

3. Contract the front of the anus and the tops of the eyeballs.

4. Contract the back of the anus and the bottoms of the eyeballs.

5. Contract the right side of the anus and the right sides of the eyeballs.

6. Contract the left side of the anus and the left sides of the eyeballs.

This exercise not only strengthens the eyes but also the pituitary and pineal glands and the inner ear, including the ear drum and canals. When you pull the eyeballs in and upward and look toward the crown, you are exercising the upper muscles and stimulating the pituitary gland and pineal gland.

When you contract and pull in the middle of your eyeballs, you are exercising the back of the eye muscles and the inner ear.

When pulling in the outer corners of the eyes, you are strengthening the side eye muscles as well as the ear canals and the ear drums.

When pulling in the inner corners of the eyes, you are strengthening the inner side muscles, the tear ducts and the nose.

When pulling in the lower parts of the eyes, you are pressing the lower part of the ear canals and the nervous system.

### G. Learn to maintain eye contact.

Some people in eye to eye contact with other people feel nervous and frightened, and their voices become very low and hard to hear because of weak organs. Some people will look around and not look into your eyes when you talk to them. This can be caused by weakness of the gall bladder and kidneys. To improve this, you can use the Inner Smile, Six Healing Sounds and Tao Rejuvenation, plus the practice of staring.

Look at your face in a mirror for two to five minutes each day for the first week. After ten days you can begin to stare at your eyes and increase your confidence by looking at your irises. Gradually you will lose the fear of looking into other people's eyes.

## VI. Nose

The nose has several important functions. When we breathe properly through the nose and not through the mouth, the nose filters out dirt, preventing it from reaching the lungs. It also regulates the temperature of the air: when the air is too cold, the nose will warm it up first. Without this regulating action, extreme temperatures could injure the lungs, make us susceptible to upper respiratory illnesses and subject to getting colds easily. One great advantage about people who practice the Tao System is that they seldom get colds.

The nose has three meridians running through it: the large intestine, the stomach, and the Governor or back Channel. Rubbing the nose strengthens the temperature regulator, stimulates the above organs, and increases hormone secretion. In China just a few needles inserted in the nose serve as a general anesthetic for any part of the body to be operated on.

An unhealthy nose affects the personality. A thin, flat and unhealthy looking nose, or a badly shaped nose, can make you less attractive to other people. A strong nose can help you to have good Chi. The nose is the first place into which the breath of life enters.

A weak nose usually will be infected, and a lot of mucous can leak into the sinuses. A weak nose also can affect the voice. A good singer always has a good nose. Rubbing and massaging the nose will increase the Chi and will improve circulation around the nose.

### A. Bring Chi energy to the hands.

Repeat the procedure for bringing energy to your hands, contracting the front part of the anus.

### B. Nostrils

Widen the nostrils. (Figure 4–25) Using the thumb and index finger, stick them into the nostrils and move them to the left and the right and up and down for ten to twenty times. This will widen the passage of air into the lungs. This also can help your sinus problems and correct the smelling sense.

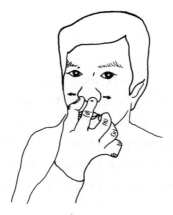

**Figure 4–25**

Widen the nostrils.

## C. Bridge

For the bridge, use your thumb and index finger and massage the bridge of your nose by repeatedly pinching it. As you do this, inhale slowly and imagine you are breathing in clean air; exhale slowly and imagine you are exhaling dirty air. Do this nine to thirty-six times. (Figure 4–26) This is effective for blocked sinuses.

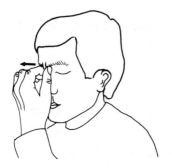

**Figure 4–26**

Massage the bridge.

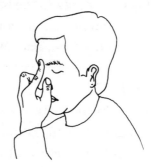

**Figure 4–27**

Massage the mid-nose.

### D. Mid-nose

For the mid-nose, place your thumb and third finger on either side of your nose, right on the bone which runs perpendicular to the nose. Place your index finger on the bridge. Inhale and press in gently. Exhale and relax. (Figure 4–27) Feel and absorb the heat from your fingers into the nose. This can increase your concentration and calm your mind.

### E. Sides of the nose

On the sides of the nose, use your index fingers, massage slowly, and gradually increase up and down the sides of your nose nine to thirty-six times. (Figure 4-28) This also helps blocked sinuses and stuffy noses. Do not do it too hard in the beginning because the sensitive tissues there are very tender and easily infected. Rub the sides of your nose up and down until you feel warm; this will help you in the cold winter and every morning when you get up.

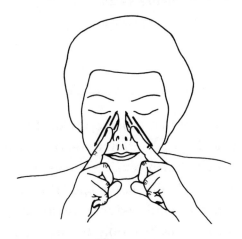

**Figure 4–28**

**Massage the sides of the nose.**

### F. Lower nose

On the lower nose, massage slowly, and gradually increase the pressure when you are sure you will not hurt yourself. Massage vigorously back and forth, using an index finger at a right angle to the nose immediately under it. (Figure 4–29) This helps blocked sinuses and stuffy, runny noses.

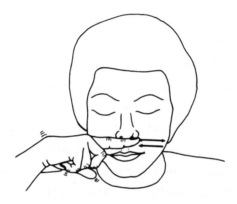

**Figure 4–29**

Massage the lower nose.

## VII. Ears

In China we believe that a person with thick, long ears will have a long, healthy life and that the personality will be more attractive. The following exercises can prevent hearing loss which occurs gradually as we age. The ears are acupuncture maps of the whole body, containing 120 points. Many acupuncturists now use only the ear points to cure many ailments as well as for weight control.

## A. Outer ear

Repeat the method for bringing energy to the hands, contracting the left and right sides of the anus.

1. Front and back: Make a space between your index and ring fingers and simultaneously rub in front and in back of the ears. (Figure 4–30(1))

2. Ear shells: Rub the ear shells with all your fingers. This will stimulate the autonomic nervous system and warm up your whole body, especially in the cold weather. (Figure 4–30(2))

3. Ear lobes: Using your thumb and index finger, pull down on the ear lobes. (Figure 4–30(3))

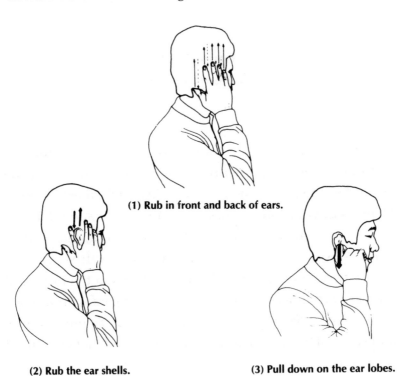

**(1) Rub in front and back of ears.**

**(2) Rub the ear shells.**

**(3) Pull down on the ear lobes.**

**Figure 4–30**

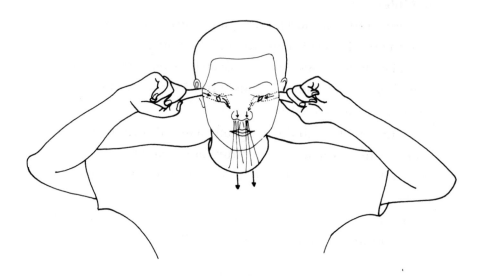

**Figure 4–31**

Outer ear drum exercise

4. Ear drum exercises: For the outer ear drum, repeat the method for bringing energy to the hands, contracting the left and right sides of the anus. Inhale and then exhale completely. Put your index fingers in your ears; it should feel as if there is a vacuum in the ears. If it does not, then exhale more. Move your index fingers back and forth six to nine times at your own pace until you can feel that the insides of the ears are moving, and pull out the fingers with a quick movement. (Figure 4–31) You should hear a "pop" sound, and you will feel that you can hear better and that your mind is clearer.

## B. Inner ear (Figure 4-32)

Repeat the method for bringing energy to the hands, contracting the left and right sides of the anus.

The inside of the inner ear, being inaccessible, is usually not exercised and grows weaker with age. These two exercises use air pressure and vibrations to strengthen the inner ear. The ear canals, the nose canal, and the mouth are connected together, so in this exercise we are using the pressure that builds in the lungs and bringing it back up to the mouth, thus adding pressure to the inner ear drums. This is how to exercise the inner ear drums.

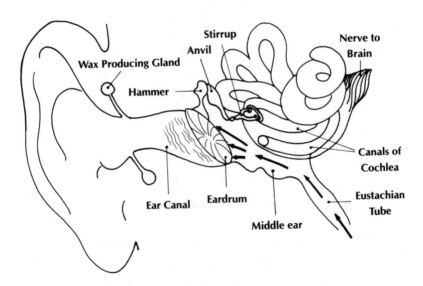

**Figure 4–32**

**Diagram of Inner Ear Drum**

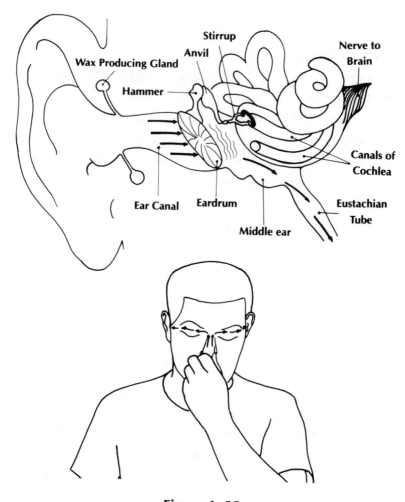

**Figure 4–33**

Inner ear drum exercise

1. Blowing exercise: Inhale, fill your lungs and nasal cavity with air, close your mouth and pinch your nostrils shut with your index finger and thumb. Blow slowly out through your closed nostrils and then swallow air. You should feel your ear drums popping. Repeat two to three times. (Figure 4–33) Do not blow too hard; they can get hurt. You must do every exercise gently for the most benefit.

2. Ear nervous system exercise: hitting the ear drum. Cover your ears with your palms, fingers pointing toward the back of your head. In this position, flick your index fingers against your third fingers so that the index fingers drum on the lower edge, or occipital bone of the skull. This will sound quite loud. The flicking of the finger that hits the bones will vibrate and stimulate the nervous system, the ears and the inner ears' mechanism. Repeat nine or more times. (Figure 4–34) The activity of the ear will be balanced and the mastoid sinus improved by this exercise.

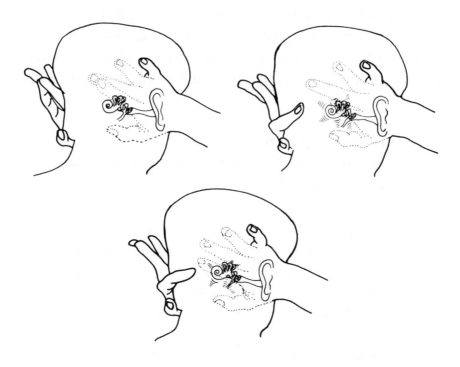

**Figure 4–34**

**Hitting the ear drum**

## VIII. Gums, Tongue, Teeth

Healthy teeth require healthy gums as their foundation. These exercises will strengthen both the gums and teeth. Teeth are the excess energy of the bones, and when the teeth get stronger, so do the bones. When the teeth and tongue are strong, your breath improves as well, eliminating bad breath.

We regard saliva as an essential form of energy which can lubricate the organs and digestive system. The tongue is the opening of the heart, and both are made of similar tissue. A healthy and clean tongue will strengthen the organs, especially the heart. You should clean your tongue twice a day with a brush or scrape it with a tongue scraper, and massage your tongue with a tongue depressor or a clean finger. Find the painful spots and massage there until the pain goes away.

### A. Bring Chi energy to the hands.

Repeat the procedure for bringing energy to the hands, contracting the middle of the anus.

### B. Gums

Open your mouth and stretch your lips tautly over your teeth. Use three fingertips (index, middle, and ring fingers) to tap the skin around the upper and lower gums. Hit around until you feel warmth in the area. (Figure 4–35)

### C. Gums and tongue

Massage your upper and lower gums with your tongue. Then suck in some saliva, press your tongue tightly against

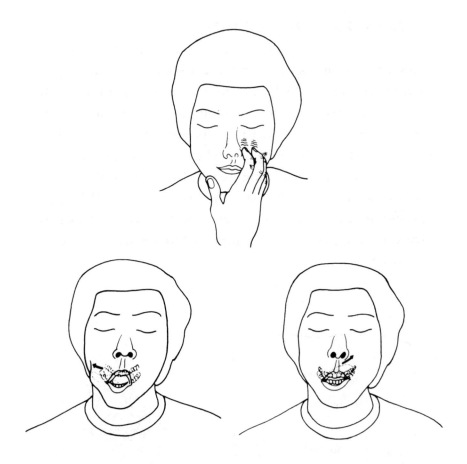

**Figure 4–35**

**Hitting the gums exercise**
**Using the tongue, massage the upper and lower gums.**

the roof of your mouth, and try to exercise the tongue. When you strengthen your tongue, you are strengthening your heart. Press around. Press the tongue to the roof of your mouth, tighten your neck muscles and swallow the saliva. This lubricates the digestive glands and organs.

### D. Tongue (Figures 4-36 and 4-37)

In a sitting position place the hands on the knees, palms down. Exhale and straighten the arms, spreading the fingers apart and keeping the hands on the knees. Open the mouth as wide as possible and thrust the tongue out and down, focused on the throat. With the tongue out as far possible, gaze at the tip of the nose. The whole body should be tense. Hold the breath for as long as you feel comfortable. Relax with inhalation and regulate the breath. This will help to strengthen the throat, the tongue and the power of speech. These exercises will help to improve foul breath and to clarify speech.

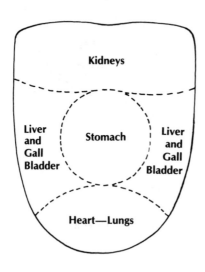

**Figure 4–36**

Diagram of tongue parts and corresponding organs

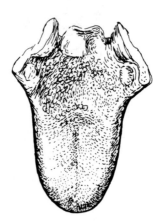

**Figure 4–37**

Tongue

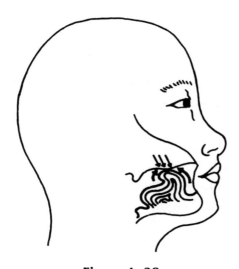

**Figure 4–38**

Press tongue to the roof of the mouth.

Inhale, then exhale as you press your tongue out and down as far as you can. Follow by pulling the tongue in and curling it. Press your tongue to the roof of your mouth as hard as you can, contracting the middle of the anus and the esophagus to help the tongue. (Figure 4–38) With more practice you will know how to use the inside force, the force from the organs, to press your tongue up. Even though the tongue has no bones to exert force, you will still be able to exercise the tongue well.

### E. Teeth clenching

Relax your lips. Click the teeth together lightly (Figure 4–39) and then clench them hard (Figure 4–40), as you inhale and pull up the middle of the anus. Do this six to nine times. Move your tongue and mouth to create a lot of saliva. The technique of swallowing the saliva is to put the tongue up to the palate and swallow quickly with a hard gulp, sending the saliva down the esophagus to your stomach. Feel the

85

saliva burn, giving out warmth to all the organs. This prevents gum disease and strengthens the teeth; it also relieves tooth aches.

### F. Energy to teeth

Close your mouth and let your teeth touch lightly. Direct the energy to your teeth. Gradually feel the electrical flow of energy there.

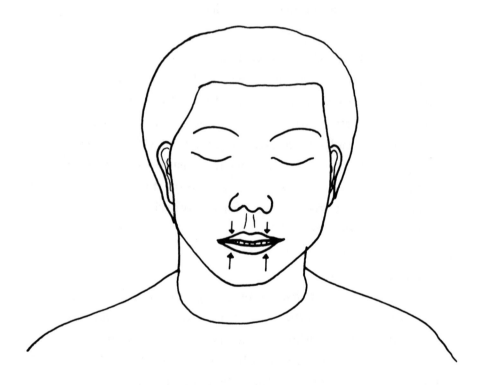

**Figure 4–39**

Click the teeth together lightly.

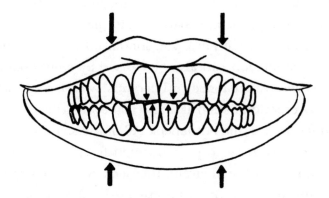

**Figure 4-40**

**Clench the teeth together hard.**

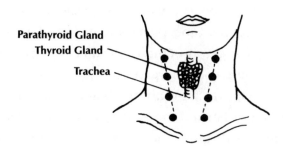

**Figure 4-41**

# IX. Neck

**A.** Thyroid and parathyroid: the site of courage, the power of speech (Figure 4-41)

The neck carries the busiest traffic in the body and is the seat of the thyroid and parathyroid glands. (Figure 4–42). When you massage here, you increase the body's metabolism. Neck tension can also be caused by emotional imbalance. When we are tense and nervous, we are responding to negative emotions, such as anger, fear and sadness. The neck is similar to a traffic bottleneck. All of the signals, as well as the emotions, have to pass through it. When under stress and under emotional strain, the neck starts to accumulate and jam the tension. Unconsciously, the neck muscles tighten, attempting to block out pain. Keeping the neck soft will help Chi flow to the higher center that is located in the brain, keeping the mind and body in harmony together.

Tension in the neck can make you less courageous. When the neck is tense, it will block self expression in the throat. With proper flow of Chi energy, we can express ourselves appropriately at the proper time, place, and in a proper way.

The neck is the passageway of many meridians and is the channel of the Chi energy of the organs. In the middle is the Governor meridian. On the sides are the bladder meridian, the triple warmer meridian and the large intestine meridian. The emotions passing through the meridians of the neck may tense and jam up there.

| Emotion: | Organ/Associate Organ: |
|---|---|
| Anger | Liver/Gall Bladder |
| Fear | Bladder/Kidneys |
| Grief | Large Intestine/Lungs |
| Hastiness | Heart/Small Intestine/Triple Warmer |
| Worry | Spleen/Stomach/Pancreas |

### B. Bring Chi energy to the hands.

Do the procedure for bringing energy to the hands and contract the front of the anus.

### C. Whole neck

Spread your thumbs apart from your other fingers. Alternate hands, rapidly wipe the neck from the chin to the base nine to thirty-six times. (Figure 4–42)

### D. Middle neck

Alternating hands, use the middle three fingers to rapidly wipe down the middle of the neck from the chin to the base nine to thirty-six times. The thyroid and parathyroid glands are in the front section of the neck. Use your thumb and the three other fingers to massage these glands. Find the painful points and massage them until you feel them open. Massaging this area will help to increase metabolism and the power of speaking.

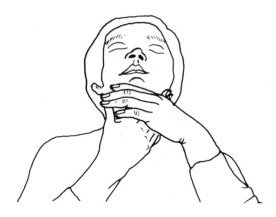

**Figure 4–42**

Wipe the neck from the chin to the base.

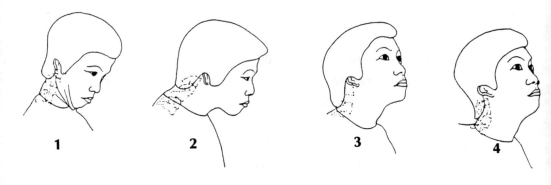

**Figure 4–43**
Turtle neck

### E. Turtle neck

Sink your chin down, then out and up. (Figure 4–43) Feel your spine press down and then expand. This will help loosen the vertebrae and discs of your neck.

### F. Crane neck

Move your chin forward, circling out, then down, then up, and out again. (Figure 4–44) Feel your spine expand and then contract.

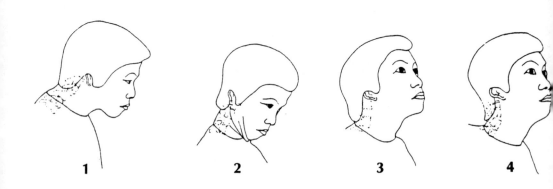

**Figure 4–44**
Crane neck

## G. Massage the neck.

Massage the points along the back of the neck and on the back along the cervical vertebrae. Start from the shoulders and go up to the base of the skull. (Figure 4–45) Use your fist to hit along the neck. (Figure 4–46) Find any painful spots and any tense spots and massage until they are released. This will greatly help to release the tension of the neck and help to detoxify the toxic accumulations in the neck area, the causes of many headaches.

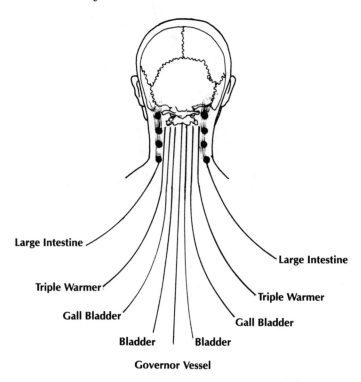

**Figure 4–45**

Massage the points along the neck.

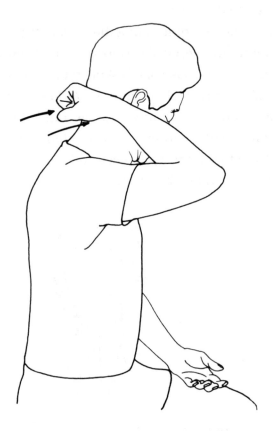

**Figure 4–46**

Use a fist to hit along the neck.

## X. *Shoulders*

Many people feel tense and worried, and their shoulders are tight and held up. The way to release the tension is by pulling up your shoulders to press against the neck, tightening the muscles of the neck and shoulders. Hold for a while, exhale deeply, and let them drop down, pulled by gravity like a sack of potatoes. (Figure 4–47) Feel the burden, worry, and stress drop down to the feet and out to the ground. Feel yourself grounded. Do this three to nine times, and the tension and worry will go away.

Relax your shoulders and chest, exhale and release more, until you feel the tenseness gone.

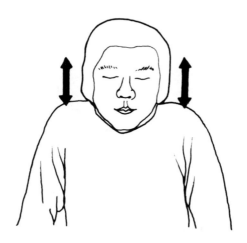

**Figure 4–47**

Dropping the shoulders will help to release tension and worry.

# 5
# Detoxifying Organs and Glands

Lightly slapping and tapping over the organs and glands help to shock the toxic sediment and increase the circulation and Chi flow to these areas. Our practitioners claim they are able to heal themselves from many chronic illnesses which are very hard to heal by conventional medicine.

## I. Thymus Gland

The thymus gland controls the immune system and is related to longevity. (Figure 5–1) Normally the thymus gland atrophies after childhood. In the higher levels of Taoist practice, the thymus gland can be regrown. This helps maintain health and vitality and supports greater spirituality. Thumbing the thymus gland can help increase the activity and release more hormones.

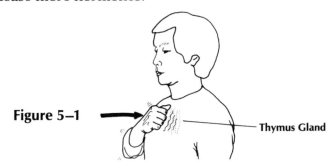

**Figure 5–1** ➡️ ——————— **Thymus Gland**

A. Bring energy to your hands by the usual procedure, contracting the front of the anus and bring the Chi toward the thymus.

B. Make a fist, inhale and thump down the middle of the upper chest from the collar bone to the nipples six to nine times. Do not talk while you are doing this or you might harm yourself.

96

## II. Heart

Lightly slapping an organ stimulates the release of toxins, which allows the organ to rebuild and repair itself. In doing these exercises, be aware that the slapping or tapping should be adjusted by you so as not to use excessive force which may be harmful.

A. Do the energy to hands procedure, contracting the left side of the anus and bringing Chi toward the heart.

B. Slap your heart lightly with your palm six to nine times. (Figure 5–2) Don't speak.

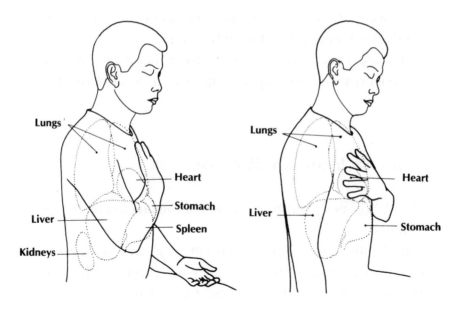

**Figure 5–2**

Slap at the heart, lungs and liver areas.

## III. Lungs

A. Bring energy to your hands, contracting the right side of the anus and bringing Chi to the lungs.

B. Using your palm, slap up and down your right lung, hitting only as hard as is comfortable. (Figure 5–2) Do not talk. Contract the left side of your anus and slap your left lung. This can help to clean out the mucous and to clean out the lungs.

## IV. Liver

A. Bring energy to the hands, contracting the right side of the anus and bringing Chi to the liver.

B. Using your palm, slap below the rib cage on the right side. (Figures 5–2) Don't speak. This can help to detoxify the liver.

## V. Stomach, Spleen, Pancreas

A. Bring energy to your hands, contracting the middle of the anus.

B. Contract the anus at the left side, and slap at the spleen, pancreas and stomach. Place one palm on top of the other and rub below the rib cage, from center to left, then left to center. (Figures 5–3 and 5–4)

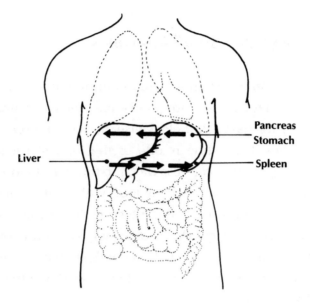

**Figure 5–3**

Rub the stomach, spleen and pancreas.

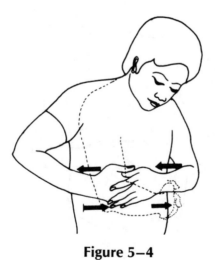

**Figure 5–4**

Rub back and forth over the liver, stomach and spleen.

## VI. Large and Small Intestines

A. Bring energy to the hands, contracting the entire anus.

B. Small intestine: With palms together, rub a small circle around your navel, first clockwise, then counterclockwise.

The small intestine is one of the longest tubes in the digestive system. A careless diet, too much hot food or dairy products, or too little fibrous food will create mucous that will stick to the walls of the intestine, block the absorption of nutrients and slow down digestion. Once mucous accumulates, it is like a snow ball that will get bigger and bigger, eventually becoming a lump which slows down the traffic of the digestive system.

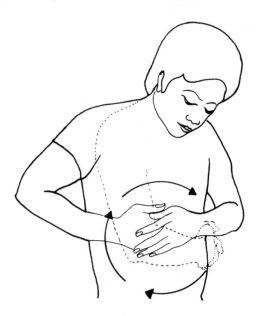

**Figure 5–5**

**Massage the abdomen.**

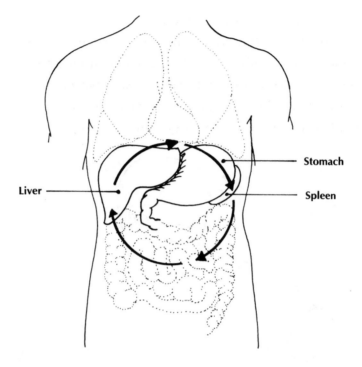

**Liver** ——————

**Stomach**

**Spleen**

**Figure 5–6**

C. Large intestine: Place one palm on top of the other and rub your abdomen in a large circle. Start on the lower right side and rub up and around in a clockwise direction. (Figures 5–5 and 5–6) This will move the energy in the intestine and relieve constipation. For diarrhea, rub counterclockwise. If you have normal elimination, rub in both directions. These exercises increase the absorption and dissolve the accumulations that stick to the large intestine's wall.

## VII. Kidneys

The kidneys act as helping to filter out waste material from the blood. If there is too much waste in the system, the kidneys cannot filter it all. The waste will tend to collect in the ducts and tubules of the kidneys, impairing their health. By hitting the kidneys' area, we shake out the harmful sediment and help prevent kidney malfunction.

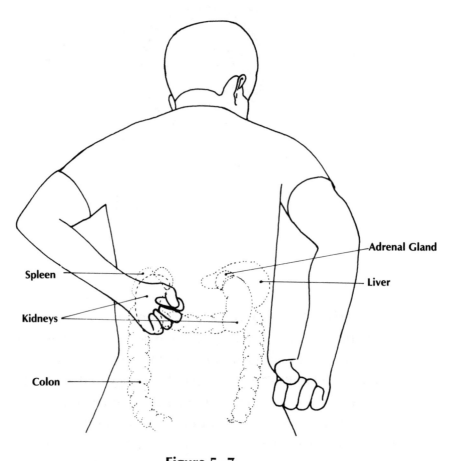

**Figure 5–7**

Hitting the kidneys will help to shake out sediment.

A. Bring energy to the hands, contracting the left and right sides of the anus.

B. Locate the kidneys just above the lowest, or floating, rib in the back on either side of the spine. Make a fist and hit the kidneys with the back of the fist between the wrist and knuckles. (Figure 5–7) Alternate hands and hit only as hard as is comfortable. This will help to shake loose the sediment, crystals, and uric acid that get caught in the kidneys. This will also strengthen the kidneys and relieve back pain.

C. Rub your hands together to warm them. Then rub your palms up and down over the kidneys until they feel warm.

## VIII. Sacrum

In the Taoist system the sacrum is regarded as extremely important. It is a pump which helps to bring spinal fluid and energy (Chi) to the brain. It is also the junction where the sexual organs, rectum, and legs meet. Sciatic pain, which shoots down the legs, originates in the sacrum; therefore, strengthening it will release this intense pain.

A. Bring energy to the hands, contracting the back of the anus to the sacrum.

B. Make a fist and use your knuckles alternately to hit both sides of the sacrum. First hit in the area of the eight sacral holes, and then the hiatus, the depression at the bottom of the sacrum. (Figure 5–8)

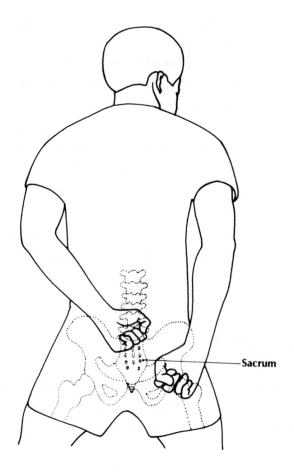

Sacrum

**Figure 5–8**

Hitting the sacrum can help in strengthening the sciatic nerves.

# 6
# Knees
# and
# Feet

## I. Knees Are Toxin Collectors, Too.

Toxins tend to collect in the lower limbs because of the slowdown of the circulation due to gravity. The most common places are the back parts of the knees. Slapping at these places will break down the toxins. The body will then eliminate the toxins out of the body by urine, bowel movements and sweat.

### A. Bring Chi energy to the hands.

Bring energy to the hands; do no contractions.

### B. Behind the knees

Prop your leg up on a chair or low table so the knee is straight. Then slap smartly behind the knee nine to eighteen times. (Figure 6–1) Although it hurts, it is extremely beneficial in releasing toxins which accumulate there. This release

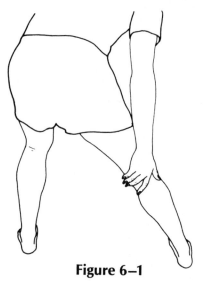

**Figure 6–1**

Slapping smartly behind the knee helps to release toxins.

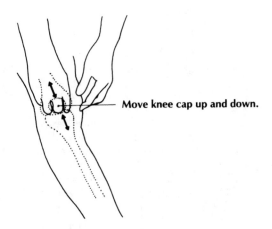

Move knee cap up and down.

**Figure 6–2**

may be indicated by the appearance of a purple dot. Use discretion as to how hard you slap, since it can be overdone. Repeat this exercise on the other knee.

### C. Knee cap massage

Massage the knee cap until it is warm. There is very little blood flowing to it and it tends to be quite vulnerable. This practice strengthens it. Massage the other knee cap.

### D. Move the knee caps

Relax the knee caps, then move them up and down to the left and right and around both clockwise and counter-clockwise. (Figure 6–2)

### E. Massage the knees

Falling down is often caused by weak knees. Massaging the knees will improve your stability and flexibility.

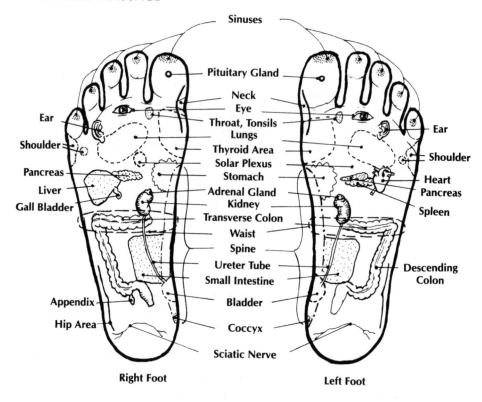

Sinuses

Pituitary Gland

Neck
Eye
Throat, Tonsils
Lungs
Thyroid Area
Solar Plexus
Stomach
Adrenal Gland
Kidney
Transverse Colon
Waist
Spine
Ureter Tube
Small Intestine
Bladder
Coccyx
Sciatic Nerve

Ear
Shoulder
Pancreas
Liver
Gall Bladder

Appendix
Hip Area

Ear
Shoulder
Heart
Pancreas
Spleen

Descending
Colon

Right Foot                    Left Foot

### Figure 6–3

**Feet are the reflexes of the whole body's organs, glands and limbs.**

## II. Feet, the Roots of the Body

Strong feet and tendons increase your stability by connecting you to the healing energy of the earth. Feet are the reflexes of the whole body's organs, glands and limbs. (Figure 6–3) They are like remote controls. Massaging will help to stimulate the organs and glands and increase the circulation.

### A. Bring Chi energy to the hands.

Bring energy to the hands; do no contractions.

## B. Massage the feet.

Take off your shoes and stockings and massage the tops and bottoms of each foot with your thumbs and fingers. Be sure to massage the kidney point, the sore spot in the center between the ball of each foot and the adjoining pad. (Figures 6–4) If you are in a hurry, massage the whole of each foot once by rubbing the sole of the foot vigorously and carefully across the top of the other foot, going from the heel to the arch to the toes. The soles of the feet have energy meridians to the entire body. Massage the feet, and when you find painful points massage them until the pain goes away. This will help to clear any blockage of Chi channel flow.

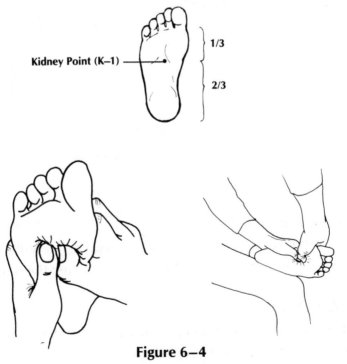

**Figure 6–4**

Massage the Kidney Point (K–1).

### C. Spread out the toes.

Spread out and separate all the toes, especially the little toes, and then release. Repeat six to nine times. This is especially good for the tendons of the feet. (Figure 6–5)

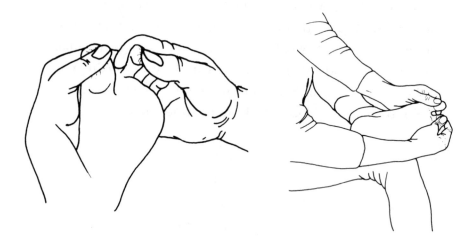

**Figure 6–5**

Separate all the toes by spreading them out.

### D. Big and second toes

Rub the big toes and second toes together rapidly. This is a good exercise to do at odd moments during the day.

### E. Rub feet together

Keep the feet warm by rubbing them together. This will help to stimulate all the body's organs.

# 7
# Constipation

## I. A Major Cause of Stress

Constipation is a major cause of stress. The key to good health is a clean colon. Much of the health field believes that as much as ninety percent of diseases are due to constipation and unhealthy colons.

The modern life that we live in—the concrete jungle, in which we eat refined foods, less fiber, more meat, less greens, less fresh fruit and fresh vegetables—causes us to have less Chi. The Chi pressure that moves the fluids and all systems in the body is lessened. Therefore, the stomach does not have enough Chi to digest food; and the small intestine will be slow in absorbing the nutrients; and the large intestine and rectum will not have enough pressure to push the waste material out. When this material stays in the colon, the body reabsorbs toxins from the waste. These reabsorbed toxins first affect the liver which, as it becomes filled with the toxins, produces negative emotions, such as anger, bad moods, and anxiety. The next to be affected is the blood which, as it becomes filled with waste material and toxins, disturbs the other organs' functions, lessening their ability to do their work, and causing stress and nervousness.

## II. Constipation Causes Holding Back and Lack of Openness.

People who hold back, are stingy and cannot let go always retain all kinds of unnecessary garbage. This type of person keeps problems inside and becomes emotional easily. This can be caused by long term constipation.

The way to overcome this kind of constipation is to try to solve problems every day and speak out in a nice way, so that the Chi that is stuck in the organs can flow. Many people today learn how to speak out but do so in a way that is not nice. This causes more problems and more constipation. Having peace of mind will permit you to solve problems in peace, letting you speak out in a nice way.

## III. Constipation Makes You Age Faster.

All toxins that are retained will collect in your body: in your skin, making it coarse, not smooth; in the neck and shoulders area, resulting in headaches and shoulder pain; and in other places. They will cause a hardening of the whole system.

The nice feeling of a clean colon will make Chi flow and will help your whole day to be pleasant, open and happy.

## IV. Abdominal Massage—the Wonder of Healing

Abdominal massage is one of the best ways to solve constipation. In the beginning you might see black and cloudy colored bowel movements during elimination. This means that long term matter stuck to the walls of the intestines has finally loosened.

When you feel the need to go to the toilet, just go. Many people like to hold back until, after a while, the feeling of the bowel is gone. As a result, they have to hold it for the next time or the next day. It should become a habit to have a bowel movement every day; the morning is the best time.

You can do the abdominal massage right before you go to sleep and right after you get up. Usually shortly after you massage in the morning you will go to the toilet to move out the bowels.

### A. Sleep face up.

Sleep face up, pull up your feet and place them your shoulders' width apart.

### B. Rub your hands until warm.

Rub your hands until warm, then rub the large intestine and the rectum, starting from the lower end of the left side up and across to the right side and down to the lower right side. (Figure 7–1) Massage in a clockwise direction for nine to eighteen times. If you feel a painful part or a knot, spend some more time massaging until it softens. Use your mind to help guide the Chi flow, according to the movement of the large intestine flow.

### C. Massage the small intestine.

To massage the small intestine, divide the abdomen into three parts. (Figure 7–2) Massage from the left line to the right line. Use the middle and index fingers and massage in a circular movement, up, down, and up, and go to the next

114

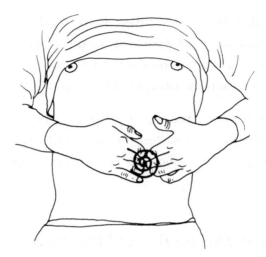

**Figure 7–1**

Massage from the lower end of the left side, up and across to the right side and down to the lower right side.

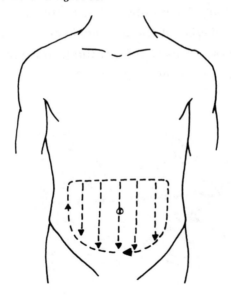

**Figure 7–2**

Divide the abdomen into three parts.

line. Repeat three to nine times. If you find a painful point or knots, massage clockwise and counterclockwise until the pain or knots are gone. Be cautious if you have had an abdominal operation; do only what you can withstand.

If you find a big lump, put your palm over it and sleep with it there; this will soften the knot and release the pain and will help you to move your bowels more easily the next day.

## V. Massage During Bowel Movements.

After you first move the bowels and stop and are waiting for the next movement, you can massage the abdomen to help clean out any "stew" that still is in the ascending colon, by rubbing clockwise at the ileocecal valve at the right side near the hip bone. Massage from the lower end of the right corner up to the rib cage. (Figure 7–3)

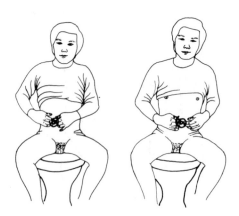

**Figure 7–3**

**Massage the abdomen during bowel movements.**

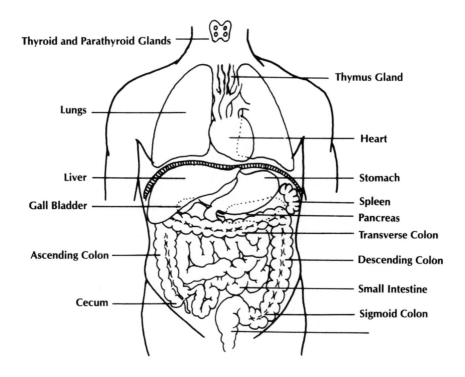

**Figure 7–4**

Massage the sigmoid colon.

Massage the sigmoid colon at the left side of the pelvis. Massaging this part can help you clear out more of the remaining "stew". (Figure 7–4)

In Tao we say that when you move the bowels, in order to be clean you must first urinate and then have the bowel movement. Finally, clean out with more urination and you will feel clean.

# 8
# Daily
# Practice

First line prevention is best. The goal of the Tao principle is to walk through to the end of life without sickness. We see that going to hospitals, entering mental hospitals, and visiting doctors and psychologists are common things. The largest part of our budgets today is for health care. The unusual thing, which can become big news, is when you see a healthy, strong old man or old woman who can walk and do things as he or she wishes, with no need to take pills and no use for Medicare. These healthy old men and women can be every one of us, if we know how to take care of ourselves.

The results of the Tao practice have been proven for many thousands of years. Tao Masters used this practice to maintain a high level of energy. When you transform the negative emotions to positive emotions, you have the power to heal yourself. If you want to get through negative states, you need to make up your own mind to set aside time and make this practice a part of your life. Invest in your own health. Make it a routine to do this every day, just like brushing your teeth and eating are necessities in your life. Don't worry about the results, simply keep practicing what you think is right for you. One day you will see the miracle happen. You will seldom catch a cold and you will hardly remember your doctor's name. Your medicine box will be empty. You will be healthier than ever before. You will accomplish more work while becoming less emotional.

## I. Warm Up In the Morning.

The Taoist tradition says to open your heart first before you open your eyes. (Figure 8–1) When you wake up, do not

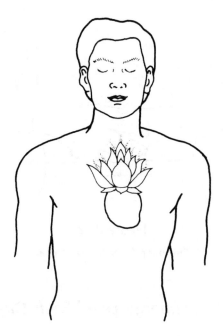

**Figure 8–1**

Before you open your eyes, open your heart.

jump out of bed and do not open your eyes. In the Taoist system we believe that all organs have souls and spirits. When we are asleep, the souls and spirits are at rest, too. They take a while to be awakened, and if you are too hasty, you can hurt them. As we say, when you are too hasty, you are hurting the energy of the organs. If you have a good morning warm up, the whole day will run smoothly.

121

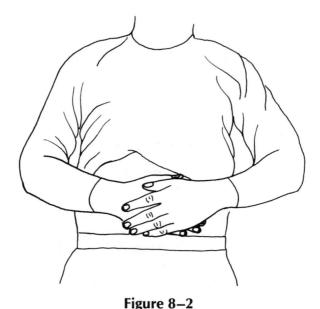

**Figure 8–2**

Put your palm on the navel area.

## II. Check Your Energy Level Each Day.

Do not open your eyes. Put your palm on the navel area. (Figure 8–2) Men, put the right palm on the navel with the left palm over it. Women, put the left palm over the navel and the right palm on top. Concentrate on your navel until you feel it become warm.

## III. Start With the Inner Smile. (Figure 8–3)

If you can, get in touch with the Inner Smile; feel the flow of it; and guide the smile all the way down from the face to the neck and through the heart, lungs, liver, kidneys, pancreas, spleen and sex organs.

Smile into the Second Line, the digestive system, and the Third Line, the nervous system and spinal cord. Smile to them and sense when the smile can get through. Keep on smiling until the pain and tension go away.

If one day it is hard to get the smile energy flowing, that means your energy levels—physical, emotional, and intellectual—are in a low cycle. Be very careful on that day, because you are in the low cycle of your biorhythm and astrologic charts. When you are too low with energy, you are likely to get yourself into trouble and have accidents. By practicing the Inner Smile and Microcosmic Orbit well, you can eventually overcome the biorhythm and astrologic charts. Spend a little bit more time in practice until you feel your smiling energy increase and flow through the organs faster. That indicates you are raising up your energy level, and the emotions can thus be controlled. Misfortune and accidents can be overcome or avoided.

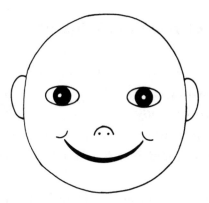

**Figure 8–3**

Start your day with the Inner Smile.

## IV. Clean Out the Blocked Energy Every Day.

If you smile through the organs and you feel obstructions and blockages in particular organs, take a little more time. Concentrate your awareness by smiling to that place where there is a blockage, until it starts to clean up. Disease always begins with the blockage of energy flow to an organ or gland and major pathway. When the energy has to flow through a major organ or gland but there is blockage, the organ starts to get less energy, less blood flow and less nutrition. Over a long period of time the organ and gland will work less effectively or not at all. No equipment can check you out as accurately as your own flow of Chi energy. When doctors find an illness, at that time an organ may be functioning at only ten percent efficiency. With a daily check-up using the Microcosmic Orbit, you can correct, maintain and strengthen yourself each day without spending much time.

## V. Clean Out Yesterday's Toxins.

The most important key to keeping healthy is to eliminate tension, worry and toxins every day so that they do not accumulate in the body. (Figure 8–4) Many people experience getting up in the morning as the hardest thing to do. They feel down, sluggish and in a bad mood with pains and aches all over.

This is the result of the accumulation of too many toxins in the body. Abdominal massage is the best way to clear the toxins out. The abdominal massage can help to release the blockages and break out the sediment every day. In the beginning some people might feel like vomiting when they hit a painful spot. This is because the toxins are starting to clear out and the organ is moving back to the proper place.

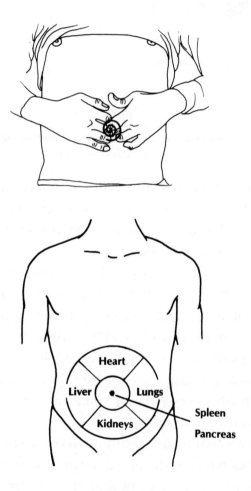

### Figures 8–4

**The major key to maintaining good health is to eliminate tension, worry and toxins every day.**

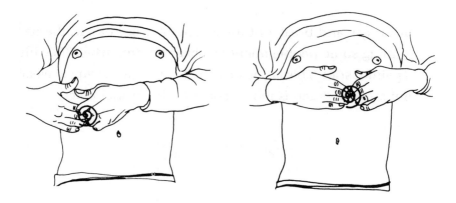

**Figure 8–5**

Massage around the navel; feel for knots or lumps;
massage to move the toxins out.

People who have had operations on the stomach or intestines have to be very careful in doing the abdominal massage. If you feel pain in the area of the operation, you might have to rub with your palm.

When you massage around the navel area and feel knots or lumps move around (Figure 8–5), that can be a bowel movement that has hardened and remained in the colon wall. If you massage and move the toxins, they will move out of their position to the rectum. People with weak energy who do not exercise the abdomen do not have enough energy to push the bowel movement up the ascending colon or push down to the rectum.

Constipation is the first thing to block energy flow, leading to back pain, headache, stomach ache and colon cancer.

Some people might not find enough time to do this in the morning, but do as much as you can manage and then massage the rest when you are at the toilet. Also, do some abdominal massage before you go to sleep.

# VI. Increase Lower Limb Circulation.

When we are asleep, the circulation slows down, especially in the legs which are the farthest away from the heart, and the toxins start to settle in the legs and feet areas. Massaging these areas can help to clean out the tension, worry and toxins that accumulated from yesterday.

As we know, the feet are the remote controls of the organs and glands. By massaging the feet, we can stimulate the organs and glands. The toes are the end and beginning of the two meridians. The outer corner of the toes is the liver meridian, which is the major detoxifying organ. When activated it will help to clear out the toxins that accumulate in the limbs and the backs of the knees.

The inside corner is the spleen meridian, which can help the immune system and help in digestion.

Practice: Lying on a bed, rub the big toe and the second toe back and forth against each other, twenty to thirty times, and feel the Chi and circulation increase. (Figure 8–6) Do it on both feet. This exercise can help to prevent hardening of the veins and arteries.

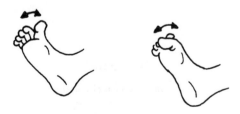

**Figure 8–6**

Move the big toe and the second toe to rub against each other back and forth.

## VII. Activate Vein Circulation. (Figure 8–7)

Veins are the return routes of the blood to the heart. The most common places for blood to clot are the veins of the feet. This can be caused by wearing high heels, wearing tight shoes, or wearing the wrong shoes. These will tend to harden the veins and slow down the entire foot circulation.

Practice:

1. Males: Start with the right foot, then the left foot, with the leg bending the feet inward toward the stomach, and exert force on the heels. Hold for a while and relax.

2. Females: Start with the left foot; then do the right foot.

If you do this exercise and feel cramping, use your fingers to pull the toes and bend them upward, or pull the toes downward until the foot recovers from the cramp.

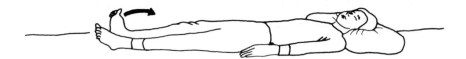

**Figure 8–7**

**Activate the vein circulation.**

# VIII. Stretch the Tendons.

When we are asleep, the tendons are at a resting stage, not stretched out. When we get up, our body feels stiff and hard to move or bend. There are thousands of stretches possible; we can spend a lot of time stretching. If you do just a few right, you can stretch all the tendons, save time and prevent yourself from being afraid to do them because you do not have enough time.

The feet, toes, hands and fingers are the ends of the extremities where all the tendons and ligaments join together. When we feel stiff, hardening starts from the extremities. Another area is the spinal cord which may tighten with its connections of many tendons and ligaments.

The extremity, and thus the main connection, of all the tendons is the tongue.

Practice:

1. Lying on your back, bend your back like a bow and stretch your hands and fingers to bend the feet and toes. Spread and stretch out the fingers and toes as far as you can, and begin to do bellows-breathing: exhale and move the stomach until it is flat and touches the spine; inhale until the stomach is inflamed. (Figure 8–8) Gradually increase the speed for about ten to fifteen times. At the final exhale, exhale deeply and stretch out your tongue as long as you can toward the chin. (Figure 8–9) Direct your eyes to look at the tip of your nose. You can repeat this two to three times. The resting period is very important. Relax your body muscles totally, and enjoy the flow of Chi energy throughout the whole body.

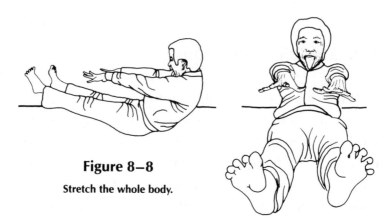

**Figure 8–8**

Stretch the whole body.

2. Bend down; use your thumbs and index fingers to hold the big toes of both feet. This will energize the liver and spleen meridians. Hold the toes and feel the energy from the thumbs go to the lungs meridian and from the index fingers to the large intestine, which is connected to the liver and spleen meridians. (Figures 8–10 and 8–11) Start to use bellows-breathing; start slowly and gradually increase it until you feel the tendons and the spinal cord get tense, and then release. After you finish you can shake the feet and slap

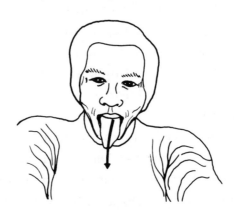

**Figure 8–9**

Stretch the tongue.

them a few times to loosen them. If you can't touch the feet, you can hold the back of the knees, calves and ankles. This will increase and activate the bladder, lungs and large intestine meridians.

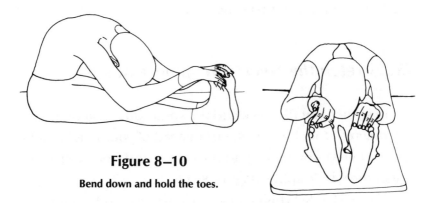

**Figure 8–10**

**Bend down and hold the toes.**

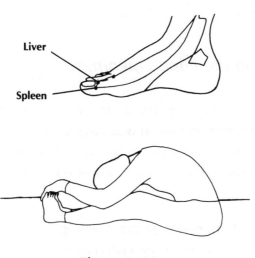

**Figure 8–11**

**Stretch the tendons exercise**

When you are more stretched, you can move to the ankles through which the bladder, stomach, liver and spleen meridians pass. Hold your ankles and feel the heat of your hands pass to the meridians.

When you can stretch more, move to touch the toes and the K–1 point, the kidneys meridian.

## IX. Stretch the Neck and Spine Tendons.

To stretch out the neck and the spine, do the same, bending down to touch the feet, but instead of your head touching the knees, you look up to the ceiling and feel the stretching of the whole spine. (Figure 8–13)

Get up slowly. When you are ready to rise, roll your body slowly to the left side and sit up; then gradually stand up and walk.

## X. Clean the Nine Openings.

We have many openings in our bodies. Taoists say we have two doors and seven windows, which are the openings that permit us contact with the outside world. These openings are able to let various kinds of pollution enter or block them out.

### A. The front door—the sexual opening

The sexual organ is regarded as the front door, which is the door of the creative life-force energy. By knowing how to control and seal it tight, the life-force energy will last longer.

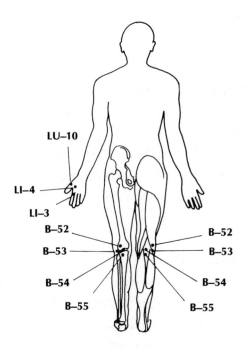

LU–10

LI–4

LI–3

B–52                              B–52

B–53                              B–53

B–54                              B–54

B–55                              B–55

### Figure 8–12

Diagram of meridians on the leg

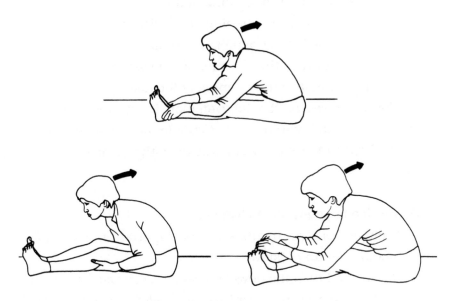

### Figure 8–13

Stretch the neck and spine tendons.

## B. The back door—the nutrients opening

The anus is regarded as the back door, which controls nutrition. Many people are not aware of what to eat and the body cannot absorb their food. They end up losing most of the nutrients to their toilets. The most expensive piece of equipment in your house can end up to be the "golden toilet".

## C. The seven windows

The two eyes, two ears, two holes of the nose, and one mouth are the seven windows. The windows are important to receive and transmit information. If a window is dirty and not strong, it will not receive information well and will not seal the life-force within.

We regard these windows as the openings of the organs.

The eyes are the opening of the liver.

The ears are the opening of the kidneys.

The nose is the opening of the lungs.

The mouth is the opening of the spleen.

The tongue is the opening of the heart.

The exercises of Tao Rejuvenation in the morning are very important. If you have the time, do more. Use the bathroom if you can, or find room outside of the bathroom to do them.

## D. Routine large intestine cleaning

Daily bowel movements are very important in reducing the accumulation of "stew" in the body.

When you finish the bowel movement, use water to clean yourself. If this is inconvenient, use toilet paper that has been wet with water and clean out the anus. Massage the coccyx and around the anus. The anus region has many arteries and veins, which are easily clotted and can become hemorrhoids. Massage the whole region 50–100 times. This is of great help in preventing or healing hemorrhoids, while helping to detoxify any accumulation in the lower region.

Knowing how to move the bowels is equally as important as eating.

## XI. Clean Out the Parts of the Face.

### A. Eyes

If you have the time, do the Tao Rejuvenation. Of all the senses' exercises, the eye exercises are my favorite.

Daily maintenance is the best prevention. Many times we do not pay much attention to the things that are close to us, like the water and air or our faces and eyes.

Many people wash their faces, but seldom wash their eyes. When working outside all day, very small particles of dust and all kinds of fiber get into the eyes and clot the tear ducts. Be sure to massage the tear ducts.

Wash the eyes with cool, clean or boiled water. Use a bowl in which you can immerse your face. Open your eyes and move the eyes around. Get all the dirt and particles out. (Figure 8–14) This will also help you remain more awake.

### B. Nose

The nose is the place where the life-force of air enters. A strong and healthy nose is the key to vitality.

Right after you clean the eyes, use another bowl of water. Make sure it is clean; preferably use cooled, boiled water.

Immerse your nose and face into the water, inhale the water into the nostrils just enough, and force it out. In the beginning you might sniff or inhale too deeply, which will cause you to cough. When you are well-practiced, the water will enter your nose and come out your mouth.

If you have difficulty handling both nostrils at one time, you can use your finger to close the right nostril while cleaning the left nostril, and then close the left nostril while cleaning the right nostril.

In the beginning you might feel pain or unpleasantness, because the nose is like a chimney—if you never clean out the smoke, it will collect there.

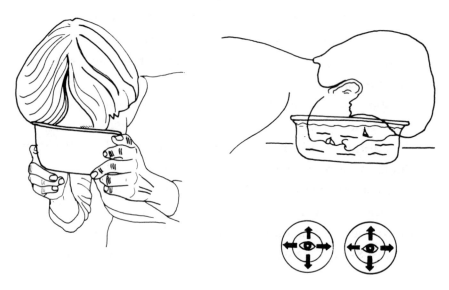

**Figure 8–14**

Clean out the eyes, nose and face.

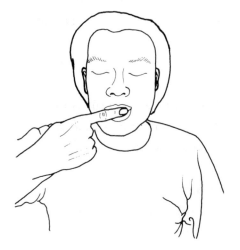

**Figure 8–15**

Massage the teeth and gums with coarse salt.

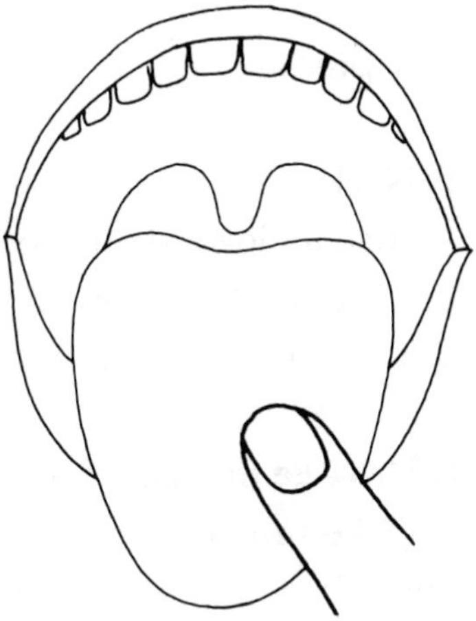

**Figure 8–16**

Massage the tongue using a clean finger
or tongue depressor.

### C. Teeth

Massaging the teeth and the gums with coarse salt is very useful. (Figure 8-15) Using your finger, touch the salt and rub the teeth and gums. Make sure that your finger is clean and the nail not too long. Massage and rub the inside and outside of the gums. Weak gums are the cause of much tooth decay. If you have time, do the teeth and gum exercises.

Massaging the tongue is very important, too. (Figure 8–16) Please see the section on tongue exercise (Chapter 4).

### D. Ears

Cleaning and exercising the ears will make you more alert and prevent hearing loss.

137

Use a clean, damp towel; rub and massage the ears, both the shells and the inner ears. See the ear exercises' section (Chapter 4).

### E. Neck

Use a clean, damp towel and rub the neck until you feel the heat and Chi flow in the neck. The neck may reveal your age; a wrinkled neck might make you look old.

### F. Massage the head and comb the hair.

Take time to massage the head and comb the scalp carefully. This can be an enjoyable moment.

## XII. Massage the Feet.

Using a towel, rub and massage your feet. Rub until you feel the feet are warm and that the Chi flows.

## XIII. Look at Yourself in the Mirror.

We know that we need to use a mirror when combing our hair. Women use mirrors most often, for make-up.

In Taoism we use the mirror to look at our own character, personality and the future. We can see what is going to happen today and how we are doing today. To foresee the future is not easy; it takes time to learn. We can see how happy we are, physically and emotionally, what is wrong with our organs and what is wrong with our senses. The face and sense organs will reveal what is inside.

If you discover that you are looking old, maybe that will stimulate you to do something for yourself.

Look in the mirror at your face. Is it arrogant, angry, sad, depressed, or fearful? Try to change the expression to a happy, joyful, smiling face. Watch the corners of your mouth. If dropped down, massage them up. Do the face massage by first warming the hands and then massaging.

## XIV. Clean Water As a Cleanser

Drinking water in the morning one to two hours before breakfast is the best for clearing out the system and providing prevention. Water can help you clean out the dirt and toxins that remain in your digestive tract. Morning is the best time to clean out.

Drink clean water. In some places you might need to boil it. Drink two to four glasses. In the beginning it might be hard to drink a lot of water. After you drink, you need to move, either walking, jogging or jumping. After that you have to do the abdominal massage to move the water around to rinse and clean out the toxins and mucous, which can move out as a bowel movement and urine.

Do not drink after a meal or before you sleep. If you drink at night, it will make you get up.

## XV. Utilize Your Time.

### A. Find time to practice.

Once the basic routine is learned, it should take only ten minutes. If you're rushed, do a few exercises, especially combing the scalp, getting a tear out, wiping the face and neck, hitting the thymus and kidneys, slapping behind the knees, and the foot rubbing massage.

You will discover that you can find a lot of free time in your day in which to practice Tao Rejuvenation. You can do hand and finger massages when you have free time, such as standing in line, waiting for people, sitting in a car, driving, or reading a magazine or newspaper. You will find that these Taoist exercises will greatly help you in improving your health.

### B. Sleepiness while driving

If you feel sleepy while driving a car, use the knocking the teeth exercise, which is very helpful in making the sleepiness go away. Moving the shoulders up to tighten the neck, pulling up the anus to vitalize the kidneys, and using the pinky finger to hold the steering wheel tight to increase circulation can make you more awake while you are driving. These exercises are sure to keep you from falling asleep when you are driving a long distance.

### C. Computer operators and desk workers

For people who work at a desk or do computer work, exercising the eyes, neck and kidneys is so important. We hope companies will adopt a system in which they give all

employees ten minutes to do the Inner Smile and Tao Rejuvenation. They will see work results increase.

If you sit and watch a video screen too long, it will make
your eyes tired, so every one to two hours close your eyes
and massage the eyeballs and move the eyeballs around until you feel good.

If you sit too long, hit the kidneys and the sacrum areas.
This is an excellent exercise for you.

### D. Watching television

Many people spend a lot of time watching television. You
can utilize that watching time by doing Chi massage. Massage the hands and feet.

### E. Boots

People tend to wear boots nowadays more often, which
makes it difficult for the feet to breathe. Since no fresh air is
circulated, find some time to take them off and massage the
feet.

### F. Evening practice

In the evening before you fall asleep, find time to soak
your feet in hot water for five to ten minutes and wipe them
dry. Rub them hot, and do the Six Healing Sounds. Do each
one three times, according to the sequence for the Six Healing Sounds described in *Taoist Ways To Transform Stress
Into Vitality.*

## XVI.  Commuting Exercise

Increasingly, more and more of our time is spent in transportation—cars, buses, airplanes, subways, trains, etc.—as

well as waiting for transportation. You can use this time to do exercises and refresh yourself.

A. If you are driving, be very careful; use your own good judgment. Do not do any exercise that will disturb your eyesight or attention on the road.

B. The neck is usually the most tense and can cause nervous tension. Do the exercises while you are driving or riding, or anywhere else, when you feel tight. Inhale, pull up your shoulders to the neck, pressing into the sides of the neck, and follow by pulling your scapulae together in your back; tense the spine and scapular muscles for only a few seconds, then exhale and drop your shoulders.

C. With your hands holding the seat, pull the spine in toward the stomach and imitate a "bowl", with the chin touching the chest, and the pelvis and sacrum tucked in. Tense the back muscles for a few seconds, especially the muscles around the kidneys, and release; you will feel the nice fresh energy rise to the top and circulate down the front. Always keep your spine loose and relaxed. Let the Chi flow without obstruction.

D. Sitting on both hands, palms up, will give you a general revitalization of the whole body. Feel the Chi energy from the palms and fingers steam up through your bottom to the base of the spine. You will feel the Chi flow, and you will feel refreshed in a short time.

E. Holding the fingers will help you rid yourself of negative emotions such as worry, fear, anger, etc. Please see the section on Finger Massages.

F. Cleansing and knocking the teeth are extremely helpful in clearing your mind. When you feel dull, sleepy, or cannot think right, cleaning the teeth will help. Please see the section on Teeth.

G. Pulling up the different parts of the anus will stimulate the organs. When you feel tired or fatigued, contract the left and right sides of the anus and wrap the Chi around the kidneys. You will help to increase the kidneys' function to clean out the toxins and give you more life-force energy.

Contract the right side of the anus to stimulate the liver. This will help give you vitality and make decisions more easily.

Contract both sides of the anus and wrap the Chi around the lungs.

## XVII. Sleep Position

A. If you feel constipated, do some abdominal massage for a while before sleeping.

B. If you like to lie on your back, lie with your hands and legs straight, and lightly hold your thumb in your fingers.

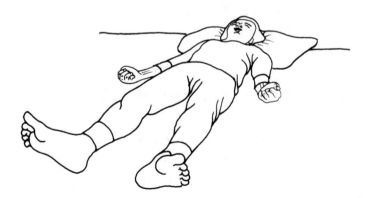

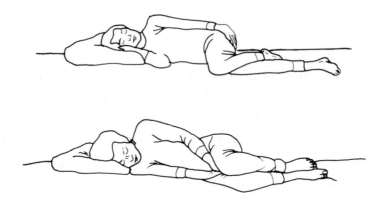

C. If you sleep on your side, try to sleep on your right side with your spine straight, your left leg bent, your right leg straight, your right hand's palm on your head but not covering your ear, and your left hand on your navel.

D. You can also lie on your side with your spine straight, curving your two legs in, and put both hands in between the legs.

E. Do not wear tight clothes. Choose a good pillow. There are many good pillows now that support the neck, not just the head, which leaves the neck hanging high in the middle.

F. Flowers in the sleeping room can make you sleep well, but do not use overly fragrant ones because they can cause you to have a lot of dreams.

## XVIII. "Oh, No! Not Another Obligation!"

The crux of any self-improvement program is continued practice. Of course, it takes a certain amount of inner discipline to practice the exercises in this book on a regular basis, preferably every day. Yet, a basic tenet of Taoism is flexibility, accommodating natural circumstances. So, be flexible with your exercise program; make it suit your individual schedule. Do as much of the routines as you have time for. If you only have time for the Lung and Kidney Sounds, do just those (but not before bed time—they are energizing when done individually). If you only have two minutes for the Inner Smile, do a quick "waterfall of smiling energy" through all the lines. Most important, try to integrate the practices into your daily life, smiling down whenever you think of it and doing the Healing Sounds when you need to relax, to deal with a particular symptom, or before bed time. Use the eye exercises after reading, writing or other close work. Get rid of a headache by doing the crown exercise, the temple massage, and bridge of the nose pinching.

The exercises are marvelous tools for relaxation and well-being, not another burdensome task to feel resentful or guilty about. Play with them and use your creativity to incorporate them into your personal life style. Make them yours. Enjoy feeling, looking, and functioning as a happier, calmer, more vital and attractive person.

# THE
# INTERNATIONAL
# HEALING TAO SYSTEM

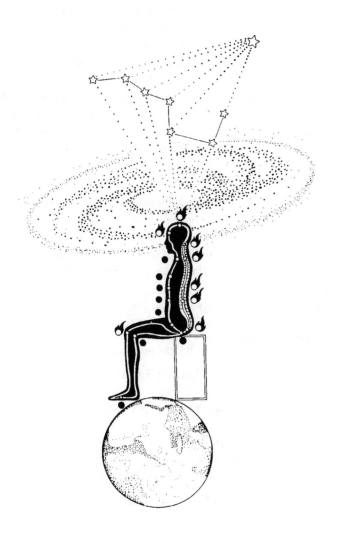

## The Goal of the Taoist Practice

The Healing Tao is a practical system of self-development that enables the individual to complete the harmonious evolution of the physical, mental, and spiritual planes the achievement of spiritual independence.

Through a series of ancient Chinese meditative and internal energy exercises, the practitioner learns to increase physical energy, release tension, improve health, practice self-defense, and gain the ability to heal oneself and others. In the process of creating a solid foundation of health and well-being in the physical body, the basis for developing one's spiritual independence is also created. While learning to tap the natural energies of the Sun, Moon, Earth, and Stars, a level of awareness is attained in which a solid spiritual body is developed and nurtured.

The ultimate goal of the Tao practice is the transcendence of physical boundaries through the development of the soul and the spirit within man.

International Healing Tao Course Offerings

There are now many International Healing Tao centers in the United States, Canada, Bermuda, Germany, Netherlands, Switzerland, Austria, France, Spain, India, Japan, and Australia offering personal instruction in various practices including the Microcosmic Orbit, the Healing Love Meditation, Tai Chi Chi Kung, Iron Shirt Chi Kung, and the Fusion Meditations.

Healing Tao Warm Current Meditation, as these practices are also known, awakens, circulates, directs, and preserves the generative life-force called Chi through the major acupuncture meridians of the body. Dedicated practice of this ancient, esoteric system eliminates stress and nervous tension, massages the internal organs, and restores health to damaged tissues.

Outline of the Complete System of The Healing Tao

Courses are taught at our various centers. Direct all written inquiries to one central address or call:

**The Healing Tao Center**
**P.O. Box 578**
**Jim Thorpe, PA 18229**

**To place orders please call: (800) 497-1017**
**Or for overseas customers: (570) 325-9820**
**Fax: (570) 325-9821**

**www.healingtaocenter.com**

## INTRODUCTORY LEVEL I: Awaken Your Healing Light

**Course 1:** (1) Opening of the Microcosmic Channel; (2) The Inner Smile; (3) The Six Healing Sounds; and (4) Tao Rejuvenation—Chi Self-Massage.

## INTRODUCTORY LEVEL II: Development of Internal Power

**Course 2:** Healing Love: Seminal and Ovarian Kung Fu.

**Course 3:** Iron Shirt Chi Kung; Organs Exercise and Preliminary Rooting Principle. The Iron Shirt practice is divided into three workshops: Iron Shirt I, II, and III.

**Course 4:** Fusion of the Five Elements, Cleansing and Purifying the Organs, and Opening of the Six Special Channels. The Fusion practice is divided into three workshops: Fusion I, II, and III.

**Course 5:** Tai Chi Chi Kung; the Foundation of Tai Chi Chuan. The Tai Chi practice is divided into seven workshops: (1) Original Thirteen Movements' Form (five directions, eight movements); (2) Fast Form of Discharging Energy; (3) Long Form (108 movements); (4) Tai Chi Sword; (5) Tai Chi Knife; (6) Tai Chi Short and Long Stick; (7) Self-Defense Applications and Mat Work.

**Course 6:** Taoist Five Element Nutrition; Taoist Healing Diet.

## INTRODUCTORY LEVEL III: The Way of Radiant Health

**Course 7:** Healing Hands Kung Fu; Awaken the Healing Hand—Five Finger Kung Fu.

**Course 8:** Chi Nei Tsang; Organ Chi Transformation Massage. This practice is divided into three levels: Chi Nei Tsang I, II, and III.

**Course 9:** Space Dynamics; The Taoist Art of Energy Placement.

## INTERMEDIATE LEVEL: Foundations of Spiritual Practice

**Course 10:**
Lesser Enlightenment Kan and Li: Opening of the Twelve Channels; Raising the Soul, and Developing the Energy Body.

**Course 11:** Greater Enlightenment Kan and Li: Raising the Spirit and Developing the Spiritual Body.

**Course 12:** Greatest Enlightenment: Educating the Spirit and the Soul; Space Travel.

## ADVANCED LEVEL: The Immortal Tao (The Realm of Soul and Spirit)

**Course 13:** Sealing of the Five Senses.

**Course 14:** Congress of Heaven and Earth.

**Course 15:** Reunion of Heaven and Man.

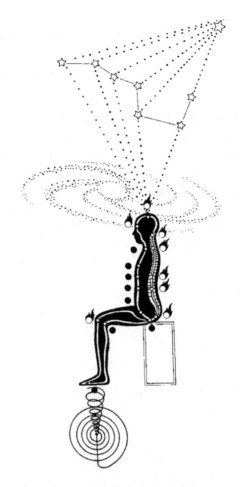

## Course Descriptions of The Healing Tao System

### INTRODUCTORY LEVEL I: Awaken Your Healing Light
### Course 1:

A. The first level of the Healing Tao system involves opening the Microcosmic Orbit within yourself. An open Microcosmic Orbit enables you to expand outward to connect with the Universal, Cosmic Particle, and Earth Forces. Their combined forces are considered by Taoists as the Light of Warm Current Meditation.

Through unique relaxation and concentration techniques, this practice awakens, circulates, directs, and preserves the generative life-force, or Chi, through the first two major acupuncture channels (or meridians) of the body: the Functional Channel which runs down the chest, and the Governor Channel which ascends the middle of the back.

Dedicated practice of this ancient, esoteric method eliminates stress and nervous tension, massages the internal organs, restores health to damaged tissues, increases the consciousness of being alive, and establishes a sense of well-being. Master Chia and certified instructors will assist students in opening the Microcosmic Orbit by passing energy through their hands or eyes into the students' energy channels.

B. The Inner Smile is a powerful relaxation technique that utilizes the expanding energy of happiness as a language with which to communicate with the internal organs of the body. By learning to smile inwardly to the organs and glands, the whole body will feel loved and appreciated. Stress and tension will be counteracted, and the flow of Chi increased. One feels the energy descend down the entire length of the body like a waterfall. The Inner Smile will help the student to counteract stress, and help to direct and increase the flow of Chi.

C. The Six Healing Sounds is a basic relaxation technique utilizing simple arm movements and special sounds to produce a cooling effect

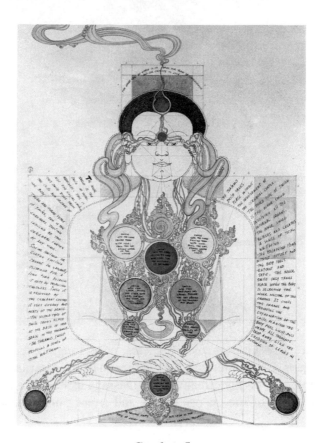

Catalog-5

upon the internal organs. These special sounds vibrate specific organs, while the arm movements, combined with posture, guide heat and pressure out of the body. The results are improved digestion, reduced internal stress, reduced insomnia and headaches, and greater vitality as the Chi flow increases through the different organs.

The Six Healing Sounds method is beneficial to anyone practicing various forms of meditation, martial arts, or sports in which there is a tendency to build up excessive heat in the system.

D. Taoist Rejuvenation—Chi Self-Massage is a method of hands-on self-healing work using one's internal energy, or Chi, to strengthen and

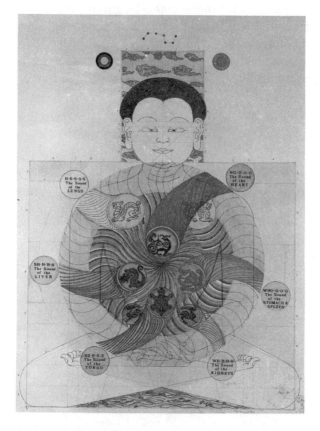

rejuvenate the sense organs (eyes, ears, nose, tongue), teeth, skin, and inner organs. Using internal power (Chi) and gentle external stimulation, this simple, yet highly effective, self-massage technique enables one to dissolve some of the energy blocks and stress points responsible for disease and the aging process. Taoist Rejuvenation dates back 5000 years to the Yellow Emperor's classic text on Taoist internal medicine.

Completion of the Microcosmic Orbit, the Inner Smile, the Six Healing Sounds, and Tao Rejuvenation techniques are prerequisites for any student who intends to study Introductory Level II of the Healing Tao practice.

## INTRODUCTORY LEVEL II: Development of Internal Power

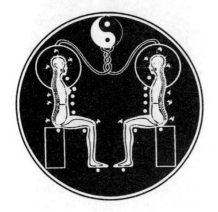

**Course 2:** *Healing Love: Seminal and Ovarian Kung Fu; Transforming Sexual Energy to Higher Centers, and the Art of Harmonious Relationships*

For more than five thousand years of Chinese history, the "no-outlet method" of retaining the seminal fluid during sexual union has remained a well-guarded secret. At first it was practiced exclusively by the Emperor and his innermost circle. Then, it passed from father to chosen son alone, excluding all female family members. Seminal and Ovarian Kung Fu practices teach men and women how to transform and circulate sexual energy through the Microcosmic Orbit. Rather than eliminating sexual intercourse, ancient Taoist yogis learned how to utilize sexual energy as a means of enhancing their internal practice.

The conservation and transformation of sexual energy during intercourse acts as a revitalizing factor in the physical and spiritual development of both men and women. The turning back and circulating of the generative force from the sexual organs to the higher energy centers of the body invigorates and rejuvenates all the vital functions. Mastering this practice produces a deep sense of respect for all forms of life.

In ordinary sexual union, the partners usually experience a type of orgasm which is limited to the genital area. Through special Taoist techniques, men and women learn to experience a total body orgasm without indiscriminate loss of vital energy. The conservation and transformation of sexual energy is essential for the work required in advanced Taoist practice.

Seminal and Ovarian Kung Fu is one of the five main branches of Taoist Esoteric Yoga.

**Course 3:** *Iron Shirt Chi Kung;*
*Organs Exercises and*
*Preliminary Rooting*
*Principle*

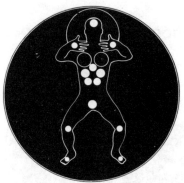

The Iron Shirt practice is divided into three parts: Iron Shirt I, II, and III.

The physical integrity of the body is sustained and protected through the accumulation and circulation of internal power (Chi) in the vital organs. The Chi energy that began to circulate freely through the Microcosmic Orbit and later the Fusion practices can be stored in the fasciae as well as in the vital organs. Fasciae are layers of connective tissues covering, supporting, or connecting the organs and muscles.

The purpose of storing Chi in the organs and muscles is to create a protective layer of interior power that enables the body to withstand unexpected injuries. Iron Shirt training roots the body to the Earth, strengthens the vital organs, changes the tendons, cleanses the bone marrow, and creates a reserve of pure Chi energy.

Iron Shirt Chi Kung is one of the foundations of spiritual practices since it provides a firm rooting for the ascension of the spirit body. The higher the spirit goes, the more solid its rooting to the Earth must be.

*Iron Shirt Chi Kung I—Connective Tissues' and Organs' Exercise:* On the first level of Iron Shirt, by using certain standing postures, muscle locks, and Iron Shirt Chi Kung breathing techniques, one learns how to draw and circulate energy from the ground. The standing postures teach how to connect the internal structure (bones, muscles, tendons, and fasciae) with the ground so that rooting power is developed. Through breathing techniques, internal power is directed to the organs, the twelve tendon channels, and the fasciae.

Over time, Iron Shirt strengthens the vital organs as well as the tendons, muscles, bones, and marrow. As the internal structure is strengthened through layers of Chi energy, the problems of poor posture and circulation of energy are corrected. The practitioner learns the importance of being physically and psychologically rooted in the Earth, a vital factor in the more advanced stages of Taoist practice.

*Iron Shirt Chi Kung II—Tendons' Exercise:* In the second level of Iron Shirt, one learns how to combine the mind, heart, bone structure, and Chi flow into one moving unit. The static forms learned in the first level of Iron Shirt evolve at this level into moving postures. The goal of Iron Shirt II is to develop rooting power and the ability to absorb and discharge energy through the tendons. A series of exercises allow the student to change, grow, and strengthen the tendons, to stimulate the vital organs, and to integrate the fasciae, tendons, bones, and muscles into one piece. The student also learns methods for releasing accumulated toxins in the muscles and joints of the body. Once energy flows freely through the organs, accumulated poisons can be discharged out of the body very efficiently without resorting to extreme fasts or special dietary aids.

Iron Shirt Chi Kung I is a prerequisite for this course.

*Bone Marrow Nei Kung (Iron Shirt Chi Kung III)—Cleansing the Marrow:* In the third level of Iron Shirt, one learns how to cleanse and

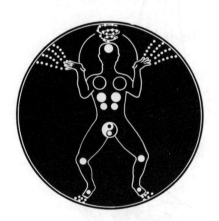

grow the bone marrow, regenerate sexual hormones and store them in the fasciae, tendons, and marrow, as well as how to direct the internal power to the higher energy centers.

This level of Iron Shirt works directly on the organs, bones, and tendons in order to strengthen the entire system beyond its ordinary capacity. An extremely efficient method of vibrating the internal organs allows the practitioner to shake toxic deposits out of the inner structure of each organ by enhancing Chi circulation. This once highly secret method of advanced Iron Shirt, also known as the Golden Bell System, draws the energy produced in the sexual organs into the higher energy centers to carry out advanced Taoist practices.

Iron Shirt Chi Kung is one of the five essential branches of Taoist Esoteric Practice.

Prior study of Iron Shirt Chi Kung I and Healing Love are prerequisites for this course.

**Course 4:** *Fusion of the Five Elements,*
*Cleansing of the Organs, and*
*Opening of the Six Special Channels*

Fusion of the Five Elements and Cleansing of the Organs I, II, and III is the second formula of the Taoist Yoga Meditation of Internal Alchemy. At this level, one learns how the five elements (Earth, Metal, Fire, Wood,

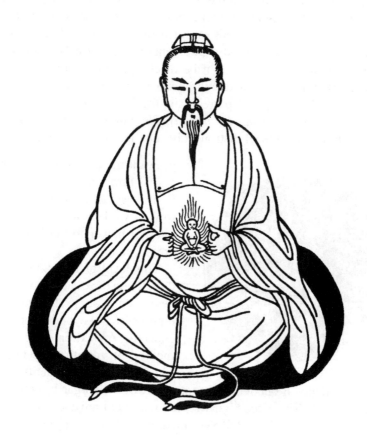

and Water), and their corresponding organs (spleen, lungs, heart, liver, and kidneys) interact with one another in three distinct ways: producing, combining, and strengthening. The Fusion practice combines the energies of the five elements and their corresponding emotions into one harmonious whole.

*Fusion of the Five Elements I:* In this practice of internal alchemy, the student learns to transform the negative emotions of worry, sadness, cruelty, anger, and fear into pure energy. This process is accomplished by identifying the source of the negative emotions within the five organs of the body. After the excessive energy of the emotions is filtered out of the organs, the state of psycho/physical balance is restored to the body. Freed of negative emotions, the pure energy of the five organs is crystallized into a radiant pearl or crystal ball. The pearl is circulated in the body and attracts to it energy from external sources—Universal Energy, Cosmic Particle Energy, and Earth Energy. The pearl plays a central role in the development and nourishment of the soul or energy body. The energy body then is nourished with the pure (virtue) energy of the five organs.

*Fusion of the Five Elements II:* The second level of Fusion practice teaches additional methods of circulating the pure energy of the five organs once they are freed of negative emotions. When the five organs are cleansed, the positive emotions of kindness, gentleness, respect, fairness, justice, and compassion rise as a natural expression of internal balance. The practitioner is able to monitor his state of balance by observing the quality of emotions arising spontaneously within.

The energy of the positive emotions is used to open the three channels running from the perineum, at the base of the sexual organs, to the top of the head. These channels collectively are known as the Thrusting Channels or Routes. In addition, a series of nine levels called the Belt Channel is opened, encircling the nine major energy centers of the body.

*Fusion of Five Elements III:* The third level of Fusion practice completes the cleansing of the energy channels in the body by opening the positive and negative leg and arm channels. The opening of the Microcosmic Orbit, the Thrusting Channels, the Belt Channel, the Great Regulator, and Great Bridge Channels makes the body extremely permeable to the circulation of vital energy. The unhindered circulation of energy is the foundation of perfect physical and emotional health.

The Fusion practice is one of the greatest achievements of the ancient Taoist masters, as it gives the individual a way of freeing the body of negative emotions, and, at the same time, allows the pure virtues to shine forth.

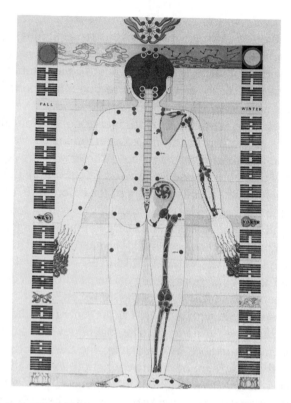

**Course 5:** *Tai Chi Chi Kung; The Foundation of Tai Chi Chuan*

The Tai Chi practice is divided into seven workshops: (1) the Original Thirteen Movements' Form (five directions, eight movements); (2) Fast Form of Discharging Energy; (3) Long Form (108 movements); (4) Tai Chi Sword; (5) Tai Chi Knife; (6) Tai Chi Short and Long Stick; (7) Self-Defense Applications and Mat Work.

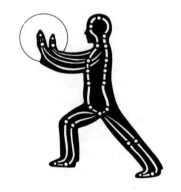

Through Tai Chi Chuan the practitioner learns to move the body in one unit, utilizing Chi energy rather than muscle power. Without the circulation of Chi through the channels, muscles, and tendons, the Tai Chi Chuan movements are only physical exercises with little effect on the inner structure of the body. In the practice of Tai Chi Chi Kung, the increased energy flow developed through the Microcosmic Orbit, Fusion work, and Iron Shirt practice is integrated into ordinary movement, so that the body learns more efficient ways of utilizing energy in motion. Improper body movements restrict energy flow causing energy blockages, poor posture, and, in some cases, serious illness. Quite often, back problems are the result of improper posture, accumulated tension, weakened bone structure, and psychological stress.

Through Tai Chi one learns how to use one's own mass as a power to work along with the force of gravity rather than against it. A result of increased body awareness through movement is an increased awareness of one's environment and the potentials it contains. The Tai Chi practitioner may utilize the integrated movements of the body as a means of self-defense in negative situations. Since Tai Chi is a gentle way of exercising and keeping the body fit, it can be practiced well into advanced age because the movements do not strain one's physical capacity as some aerobic exercises do.

Before beginning to study the Tai Chi Chuan form, the student must complete: (1) Opening of the Microcosmic Orbit, (2) Seminal and Ovarian Kung Fu, (3) Iron Shirt Chi Kung I, and (4) Tai Chi Chi Kung.

Tai Chi Chi Kung is divided into seven levels.

*Tai Chi Chi Kung I is comprised of four parts:*
a. Mind: (1) How to use one's own mass together with the force of gravity; (2) how to use the bone structure to move the whole body with very little muscular effort; and (3) how to learn and master the thirteen movements so that the mind can concentrate on directing the Chi energy.
b. Mind and Chi: Use the mind to direct the Chi flow.
c. Mind, Chi, and Earth force: How to integrate the three forces into one unit moving unimpeded through the bone structure.
d. Learn applications of Tai Chi for self-defense.

*Tai Chi Chi Kung II—Fast Form of Discharging Energy:*
a. Learn how to move fast in the five directions.
b. Learn how to move the entire body structure as one piece.
c. Discharge the energy from the Earth through the body structure.

*Tai Chi Chi Kung III—Long Form Tai Chi Chuan:*
a. Learn the 108 movements form.
b. Learn how to bring Chi into each movement.
c. Learn the second level of self-defense.
d. Grow "Chi eyes."

*Tai Chi Chi Kung IV—the Tai Chi Sword.*
*Tai Chi Chi Kung V—Tai Chi Knife.*
*Tai Chi Chi Kung VI—Tai Chi Short and Long Stick.*
*Tai Chi Chi Kung VII—Application of Self-Defense and Mat Work.*
Tai Chi Chuan is one of the five essential branches of the Taoist practice.

**Course 6:** *Taoist Five Element Nutrition; Taoist Healing Diet*
Proper diet in tune with one's body needs, and an awareness of the seasons and the climate we live in are integral parts of the Healing Tao. It is not enough to eat healthy foods free of chemical pollutants to have good health. One has to learn the proper combination of foods according to the five tastes and the five element theory. By knowing one's predominant element, one can learn how to counteract imbalances inherent in one's nature. Also, as the seasons change, dietary needs vary. One must know how to adjust them to fit one's level of activity. Proper diet can become an instrument for maintaining health and cultivating increased levels of awareness.

**INTRODUCTORY LEVEL III: The Way of Radiant Health**

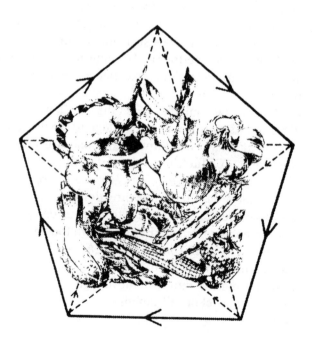

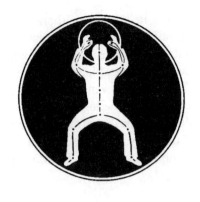

**Course 7:** *Healing Hands Kung Fu; Awaken the Healing Hand—Five Finger Kung Fu*

The ability to heal oneself and others is one of the five essential branches of the Healing Tao practice. Five Finger Kung Fu integrates both static and dynamic exercise forms in order to cultivate and nourish Chi which accumulates in the organs, penetrates the fasciae, tendons, and muscles, and is finally transferred out through the hands and fingers. Practitioners of body-centered therapies and various healing arts will benefit from this technique. Through the practice of Five Finger Kung Fu, you will learn how to expand your breathing capacity in order to further strengthen your internal organs, tone and stretch the lower back and abdominal muscles, regulate weight, and connect with Father Heaven and Mother Earth healing energy; and you will learn how to develop the ability to concentrate for self-healing.

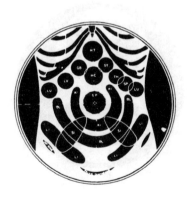

**Course 8:** *Chi Nei Tsang; Organ Chi Transformation Massage*

The practice is divided into three levels: Chi Nei Tsang I, II, and III.

Chi Nei Tsang, or Organ Chi Transformation Massage, is an entire system of Chinese deep healing that works with the energy flow of the five major systems in the body: the vascular system, the lymphatic system, the nervous system, the tendon/muscle system, and the acupuncture meridian system.

In the Chi Nei Tsang practice, one is able to increase energy flow to specific organs through massaging a series of points in the navel area. In Taoist practice, it is believed that all the Chi energy and the organs, glands, brain, and nervous system are joined in the navel; therefore, energy blockages in the navel area often manifest as symptoms in other parts of the body. The abdominal cavity contains the large intestine, small intestine, liver, gall bladder, stomach, spleen, pancreas, bladder, and sex organs, as well as many lymph nodes. The aorta and vena cava divide into two branches at the navel area, descending into the legs.

Chi Nei Tsang works on the energy blockages in the navel and then follows the energy into the other parts of the body. Chi Nei Tsang is a very deep science of healing brought to the United States by Master Mantak Chia.

### Course 9: *Space Dynamics; The Taoist Art of Placement*

Feng Shui has been used by Chinese people and emperors for five thousand years. It combines ancient Chinese Geomancy, Taoist Metaphysics, dynamic Psychology, and modern Geomagnetics to diagnose energy, power, and phenomena in nature, people, and buildings. The student will gain greater awareness of his own present situation, and see more choices for freedom and growth through the interaction of the Five Elements.

### INTERMEDIATE LEVEL: Foundations of Spiritual Practice

**Course 10:** *Lesser Enlightenment (Kan and Li); Opening of the Twelve Channels; Raising the Soul andDeveloping theEnergy Body*

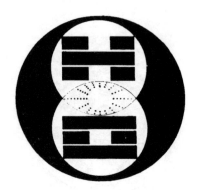

Lesser Enlightenment of Kan and Li (Yin and Yang Mixed): This formula is called *Siaow Kan Li* in Chinese, and involves a literal steaming of the sexual energy (Ching or creative) into life-force energy (Chi) in order to feed the soul or energy body. One might say that the transfer of the sexual energy power throughout the whole body and brain begins with the practice of Kan and Li. The crucial secret of this formula is to reverse the usual sites of Yin and Yang power, thereby provoking liberation of the sexual energy.

This formula includes the cultivation of the root (the Hui-Yin) and the heart center, and the transformation of sexual energy into pure Chi at the navel. This inversion places the heat of the bodily fire beneath the coolness of the bodily water. Unless this inversion takes place, the fire simply moves up and burns the body out. The water (the sexual fluid) has the tendency to flow downward and out. When it dries out, it is the end. This formula reverses normal wasting of energy by the highly advanced method of placing the water in a closed vessel (cauldron) in the body, and then cooking the sperm (sexual energy) with the fire beneath. If the water (sexual energy) is not sealed, it will flow directly into the fire and extinguish it or itself be consumed.

This formula preserves the integrity of both elements, thus allowing the steaming to go on for great periods of time. The essential formula is to never let the fire rise without having water to heat above it, and to never allow the water to spill into the fire. Thus, a warm, moist steam is produced containing tremendous energy and health benefits, to regrow all the glands, the nervous system, and the lymphatic system, and to increase pulsation.

The formula consists of:

1. Mixing the water (Yin) and fire (Yang), or male and female, to give birth to the soul;
2. Transforming the sexual power (creative force) into vital energy (Chi), gathering and purifying the Microcosmic outer alchemical agent;
3. Opening the twelve major channels;
4. Circulating the power in the solar orbit (cosmic orbit);
5. Turning back the flow of generative force to fortify the body and the brain, and restore it to its original condition before puberty;
6. Regrowing the thymus gland and lymphatic system;
7. Sublimation of the body and soul: self-intercourse. Giving birth to the immortal soul (energy body).

**Course 11:** *Greater Enlightenment (Kan and Li); Raising the Spirit and Developing the Spiritual Body*

This formula comprises the Taoist Dah Kan Li (Ta Kan Li) practice. It uses the same energy relationship of Yin and Yang inversion but increases to an extraordinary degree the amount of energy that may be

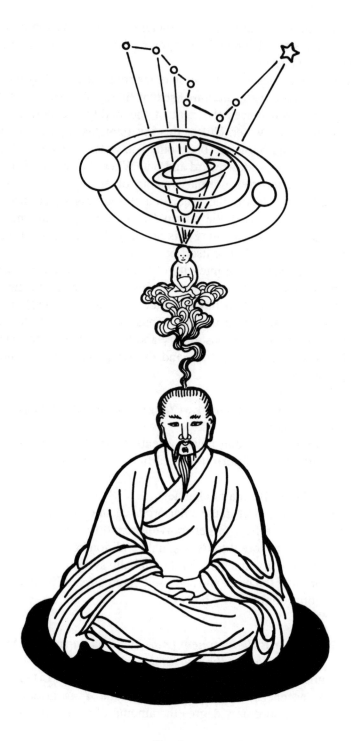

drawn up into the body. At this stage, the mixing, transforming, and harmonizing of energy takes place in the solar plexus. The increasing amplitude of power is due to the fact that the formula not only draws Yin and Yang energy from within the body, but also draws the power directly from Heaven and Earth or ground (Yang and Yin, respectively), and adds the elemental powers to those of one's own body. In fact, power can be drawn from any energy source, such as the Moon, wood, Earth, flowers, animals, light, etc.

The formula consists of:
1. Moving the stove and changing the cauldron;
2. Greater water and fire mixture (self-intercourse);
3. Greater transformation of sexual power into the higher level;
4. Gathering the outer and inner alchemical agents to restore the generative force and invigorate the brain;
5. Cultivating the body and soul;
6. Beginning the refining of the sexual power (generative force, vital force, Ching Chi);
7. Absorbing Mother Earth (Yin) power and Father Heaven (Yang) power. Mixing with sperm and ovary power (body), and soul;
8. Raising the soul;
9. Retaining the positive generative force (creative) force, and keeping it from draining away;
10. Gradually doing away with food, and depending on self sufficiency and universal energy;
11. Giving birth to the spirit, transferring good virtues and Chi energy channels into the spiritual body;
12. Practicing to overcome death;
13. Opening the crown;
14. Space travelling.

**Course 12:** *Greatest Enlightenment (Kan and Li)*

This formula is Yin and Yang power mixed at a higher energy center. It helps to reverse the aging process by re-establishing the thymus glands and increasing natural immunity. This means that healing energy is radiated from a more powerful point in the body, providing greater benefits to the physical and ethereal bodies.

The formula consists of:
1. Moving the stove and changing the cauldron to the higher center;
2. Absorbing the Solar and Lunar power;
3. Greatest mixing, transforming, steaming, and purifying of sexual

power (generative force), soul, Mother Earth, Father Heaven, Solar and Lunar power for gathering the Microcosmic inner alchemical agent;

4. Mixing the visual power with the vital power;
5. Mixing (sublimating) the body, soul and spirit.

## ADVANCED LEVEL: The Immortal Tao
## The Realm of Soul and Spirit
### Course 13: *Sealing of the Five Senses*

This very high formula effects a literal transmutation of the warm current or Chi into mental energy or energy of the soul. To do this, we must seal the five senses, for each one is an open gate of energy loss. In other words, power flows out from each of the sense organs unless there is an esoteric sealing of these doors of energy movement. They must release energy only when specifically called upon to convey information.

Abuse of the senses leads to far more energy loss and degradation than people ordinarily realize. Examples of misuse of the senses are as follows: if you look too much, the seminal fluid is harmed; listen too much, and the mind is harmed; speak too much, and the salivary glands are harmed; cry too much, and the blood is harmed; have sexual inter-course too often, and the marrow is harmed, etc.

Each of the elements has a corresponding sense through which its elemental force may be gathered or spent. The eye corresponds to fire; the tongue to water; the left ear to metal; the right ear to wood; the nose to Earth.

The fifth formula consists of:
1. Sealing the five thieves: ears, eyes, nose, tongue, and body;
2. Controlling the heart, and seven emotions (pleasure, anger, sorrow, joy, love, hate, and desire);
3. Uniting and transmuting the inner alchemical agent into life-pre-serving true vitality;
4. Purifying the spirit;
5. Raising and educating the spirit; stopping the spirit from wandering outside in quest of sense data;
6. Eliminating decayed food, depending on the undecayed food, the universal energy is the True Breatharian.

### Course 14: *Congress of Heaven and Earth*

This formula is difficult to describe in words. It involves the incarna-tion of a male and a female entity within the body of the adept. These two entities have sexual intercourse within the body. It involves the mixing of the Yin and Yang powers on and about the crown of the head, being totally open to receive energy from above, and the regrowth of the pineal gland to its fullest use. When the pineal gland has developed to its fullest potential, it will serve as a compass to tell us in which direction our aspirations can be found. Taoist Esotericism is a method of mastering the spirit, as described in Taoist Yoga. Without the body, the Tao cannot be attained, but with the body, truth can never be realized. The practitioner of Taoism should preserve his physical body with the same care as he would a precious diamond, because it can be used as a medium to achieve immortality. If, however, you do not abandon it when you reach your destination, you will not realize the truth.

This formula consists of:
1. Mingling (uniting) the body, soul, spirit, and the universe (cosmic orbit);
2. Fully developing the positive to eradicate the negative completely;
3. Returning the spirit to nothingness.

**Course 15:** *Reunion of Heaven and Man*

We compare the body to a ship, and the soul to the engine and propeller of a ship. This ship carries a very precious and very large diamond which it is assigned to transport to a very distant shore. If your ship is damaged (a sick and ill body), no matter how good the engine is, you are not going to get very far and may even sink. Thus, we advise against spiritual training unless all of the channels in the body have been properly opened, and have been made ready to receive the 10,000 or 100,000 volts of super power which will pour down into them. The Taoist approach, which has been passed down to us for over five thousand years, consists of many thousands of methods. The formulae and practices we describe in these books are based on such secret knowledge and the author's own experience during over twenty years of study and of successively teaching thousands of students.

The main goal of Taoists:
1. This level—overcoming reincarnation, and the fear of death through enlightenment;
2. Higher level—the immortal spirit and life after death;
3. Highest level—the immortal spirit in an immortal body. This body functions like a mobile home to the spirit and soul as it moves through the subtle planes, allowing greater power of manifestation.

# HOW TO ORDER

**Prices and Taxes:**
Subject to change without notice. New York State residents please add 8.25% sales tax.

**Payment:**
Send personal check, money order, certified check, or bank cashier's check to:

**The Healing Tao Center**
**P.O. Box 578**
**Jim Thorpe, PA 18229**
**To place orders please call: (800) 497-1017**
**or for overseas customers: (570) 325-9820**
**Fax: (570) 325-9821**
**All foreign checks must be drawn on a U.S. bank. Mastercard**
**Visa, and American Express cards accepted.**

**Shipping**
*Domestic Shipping* via UPS, requires a complete street address. Allow 3-4 weeks for delivery

❖ **Please call or write for additional information in your area** ❖

**www.healingtaocenter.com**

**T.A.O. - Inc. (Transformational Assistance For Offenders)**
**James Cappellano, Executive Director**
**P.O. Box 471, Revere, MA 02151**
E-mail: **taojching@msn.com**      Website: **www.tao-inc.org**

Teaching the Healing Tao to perpetrators of violence, many of who are drug and alcohol abusers, addresses the seed causes of crime and brutality. This invokes a deeper understanding of life resulting in personal transformation to a lifestyle of non-harming. It is an ideal self-help method to empower prisoners to help themselves within the confines of prison. Books and letters sent have an exponential effect with prisoners sharing the books and benefits of their practice with each other.

T.A.O. - Inc. is a non-profit organization and provides: an interactive newsletter for prisoners and instructors, a website pen-pal list, volunteer instructors and free books to inmates. The program is sustained through individual cash donations, office supplies and stamps (34¢, 55¢ & $1 are constantly needed). Contributions are tax-deductible. Please make checks payable to T.A.O., Inc. For a free copy of the newsletter please include a first-class stamp with your name and address.

# NOTES

# NOTES

# NOTES

---

# NOTES

# NOTES

# NOTES

# NOTES

# NOTES